MEDICINE, MORALS AND MAN

MEDICINE, MORALS AND MAN

EDITED BY

Dr. Ernest Claxton
M.B., B.S., M.R.C.S., L.R.C.P., D.T.M. & N.

Previously Principal Assistant Secretary of the British Medical Association

AND

H. A. C. McKay, M.A., D.SC. (Oxon)
Atomic Energy Research Establishment Harwell, Didcot, Berks.

LONDON

BLANDFORD PRESS

First published 1969
© Blandford Press Ltd.,
167, High Holborn, London, W.C.1

SBN 7137 0508 6 Hardback
SBN 7157 0509 4 Paperback

Printed by C. Tinling and Co. Ltd.,
Liverpool, London and Prescot

CONTENTS

CONTENTS

INTRODUCTION

DR ERNEST CLAXTON

'Soon G.P.'s are going to be obsolete', said the young pathologist. 'We'll feed all the results we get in the path. lab. into a computer, and the computer will give the diagnosis. We may not even bother with a diagnosis – the computer can go straight on to prescribing treatment. Unlike the G.P., the computer can never get out-of-date, because we'll always be revising the programme to include the latest discoveries. Ultimately even specialists may become redundant, though for some time to come there'll be a proportion of cases for which the computer has not been programmed.'

Is this a Utopian dream or a nightmare? Sheer pressure of work is pushing medicine towards automation. Automation certainly has a legitimate place in dealing with the routine side of medical services. But what will happen if the therapeutic value of a continuing confidence-promoting doctor-patient relationship is lost? If people become, as it were, mere punched cards in a health-welfare machine, may they not in their anxiety and frustration react by greater development of psychosomatic disorders?

It is well-known that an increasing proportion of patients need help that goes beyond physical treatment. Mental illness is on the increase, and so too are stress diseases. Hospital beds are too often filled with patients such as attempted suicides who should not be there at all. Diseases attributable largely to self-indulgence also loom large today – alcoholism, lung cancer, V.D. and drug-addiction. We have mastered most of the killer diseases and infant mortality of the past, but in their place we have reaped a new and costly crop of ill-health, and the ironical thing is that so much of it is unnecessary and preventable.

There are times indeed when one feels that our present pursuit of health, though observably most successful, is in fact a chase after an ever-receding target. We appear to be

1

caught in a vicious spiral in which sickness and accident cases multiply faster than the means of cure. We blame modern civilisation, the affluent society. A new approach to health seems to be needed, or at least a change of emphasis, and if it is true that society is partly to blame for sickness, then it follows that our new approach will need to extend from the health of the individual to the health of the community and the whole world.

The diseases that increasingly dominate the medical scene today, being disorders of mind and character, are precisely those that are least amenable to computerisation. If treatment is to be anything more than a treatment of symptoms the doctor must penetrate to the motivating forces in the patient's life. Though in some cases this calls for skilled psychiatry, there is much that the ordinary doctor can do on a person-to-person level in the course of his practice, provided he has himself found a positive answer to life's problems.

Much more in the sphere of preventive medicine is needed, if the medical services are not to be overwhelmed – and this is the responsibility of everyone. The present-day pattern of disease emphasises the truth that health depends *inter alia* on the way people live – on their habits, character, moral standards, religious beliefs if any, and aims in life. Equally the health of society is bound up with its prevailing mores and values. If something could be achieved in this realm, a new and sounder foundation for health might be laid, and what is more, a contribution might be made towards a renaissance of the human spirit.

With these considerations in mind I suggested to my brother, the Bishop of Blackburn, that we should take joint action amongst our colleagues. This took the form of a Consultation at St George's House, Windsor Castle, on the theme 'Medicine, Science and Religion and the Health of Society'. It took place in March 1968, and was attended by thirty-five people, including bishops, professors, medical consultants and others. As at other St George's House Consultations, the aim was 'to discuss areas of conflict and tension and moral uncertainty'.

In our invitation we gave as the purpose of the Consultation:

> To assess the advances in medicine in relation to the needs of mankind and to discuss the relationship of faith to problems of survival and the development of society. To explore the meaning and relevance of the Church's role to heal mankind. Medicine with its traditional methods and values finds itself practising in a different milieu from that in which its ethics and objectives were laid down. The Church similarly faced with scientific discoveries and changing mores is forced to re-examine its traditional role. The health, progress and fibre of the nation depend to a great extent on both Medicine and Religion.

The general approach we had in view was outlined as follows in a paper sent to the participants beforehand:

> Emphasis will be on preventive medicine and social health. It has been said that the major problem facing Medicine today is no longer disease but human happiness. The provision of means of health, housing, food and knowledge does not mean that they are rightly used. Man himself must be dealt with, his emotions, his attitudes and his motives. If doctors can learn from theologians how they can deal with human nature, and if theologians can understand how to communicate both with their medical colleagues and the people with whom each group is concerned, then there will be some hope of common and effective action.
>
> Science rightly used can be the medium for health and happiness but without self control, unselfish motives and conviction, people exploit it and each other, misuse its discoveries and thus endanger society.

The Consultation was a private one, and no record was kept beyond a brief summary by one of the participants who acted as rapporteur. The ideas put forward seemed to me, however, to be of sufficient importance to be given a wider dissemination. The new approach to health that I have spoken of, is evidently already partly in being. There is a need to articulate, develop and spread it.

To this end I have invited authorities in different fields to contribute their views. They are on the same general theme as the St George's House Consultation, and three of them (those by Professor F. E. Camps, Dr D. Robertson and the Rev. A. Thornhill) are directly based on papers presented at the Consultation.

It is my hope that the material in this book will show those concerned with medicine and welfare how they can go beyond their present beneficent role, how they can on the one hand put the emphasis on treating the whole person in his social environment, and on the other, how they can begin to change the social climate itself. The two things are of course closely connected. The individual is a cell in the body of society, and the health of the one is intimately related to the health of the other.

The task is not one for the medical profession alone. Other disciplines than those of medicine are increasingly recognised as being needed to achieve health, as the papers in this book make clear. The medical profession, moreover, has valid reason to concern itself with all the forces that influence the way people and society live, and to seek co-operation with, for example, parents, teachers, clergy and local authorities, and looking further afield, with the entertainment world and those who control the mass communication media.

To be effective in all this I am convinced that we must enter the realm of morals and faith. The need of men and nations is for moral and spiritual regeneration. I long to see my own profession of medicine playing its full part in creating a world not only of health but also of harmony. As doctors we cannot avoid influencing for good or ill the conduct of those we treat, nor can we escape giving a lead on many of the issues of the day. We have a high level of responsibility, and I believe that we can discharge it in unimagined ways if we find a new illumination from God. I see no reason why we should not join with others in a quiet, constructive revolution, in which people find purpose and the world finds peace.

Part One

The Present Context

1

MEDICINE'S HISTORIC ROLE

KENNETH D. KEELE, M.D., B.S., F.R.C.P., M.R.C.S.

Dr Keele is well known as a medical historian. He is Consultant Physician to the Ashford and Staines Hospitals, and Lecturer in the Faculty of the History of Medicine and Pharmacy of the Society of Apothecaries of London. In 1958 he was Visiting Professor in the History of Medicine, Yale University, and in 1966 he held a similar appointment at the University of California.

There are two main factors to be considered when talking of the historic role of medicine. First there is the nature of the practice of medicine itself which has altered vastly during the past centuries and is becoming scientific more rapidly than ever before. Second, there is the context of society within which medicine works, another factor which is also changing very rapidly under the influence of scientific discovery.

Doctor and Patient
For many centuries medicine has been regarded as the art of applying theoretical knowledge called science, to relieving the symptoms and suffering of a patient. It has been usual to look upon the medical art as being applied to the individual and not to society as a whole. The realm of a doctor has been therefore the treatment of an individual patient.

The science of medicine, that is to say the knowledge behind the healing art of practice, has varied greatly. In prehistoric days this consisted of theories in which disease depended upon the influence of divine magical external powers upon the body of the patient. It was not even considered that disease arose internally, primarily from natural disorders of the body. Thus 'intrusion bodies' as they were called, such as 'elf shots', forces of the evil eye, the actions of demons and even gods, were made responsible for the infliction of disease. Treatment consisted of the expulsion of the intrusive bodies; thus the medicine-man's role was to withdraw such bodies from the patient. Devils, imaginary arrows and so forth, were expelled from the patient's body and he then felt better, or a spell was counteracted by the greater powers of the medicine-man. It might justly be said that this was the period of complete ignorance regarding the organic nature of internal diseases. This criticism does not apply to surgery, which from earliest times was more influenced by commonsense; for example when a limb was broken it was set in a splint. Wounds were closed and dressed.

In this context it is easy to see how disease came to be looked upon as punishment for sin by a righteous and angry god. In this phase of civilisation the gods, and indeed God himself, played a large part as the cause of plagues and epidemics, as is to be seen in the Old Testament. This was logical, given the theories upon which the premises were built. In fact it is Babylonian medicine which we see practised by Jesus in the New Testament in the casting out of devils and the healings by faith that He performed. This kind of medicine continued throughout the world in all the great early civilisations and it continues still where societies preserve the outlook of the ancient Egyptians or Babylonians. But it is present, too, wherever the psychosomatic element in disease is recognised.

This outlook was altered by the Greeks who introduced objective speculative theories of disease. They also introduced an objective method of acquiring a science of medicine, which was the work of Hippocrates and his school. Just as the Greeks postulated the four material elements, earth, air, fire and water as the basis of all things, so they postulated equally speculative causes of disease which depended on the qualities of the four elements, viz. heat, cold, dryness and wetness; and also on the balance of the humours, blood, black bile, yellow bile and phlegm. These hypothetical factors were developed into an extremely complex theory of disease. The most notable exponent of this was the great physician Galen who lived in the reign of the Roman Emperor Marcus Aurelius, between A.D. 150–200. Galen not only enunciated speculative theories of disease, but founded treatments upon these theories, and these came right down in history, being practised in Europe as recently as the beginning of the nineteenth century.

Why was it that there was no 'real' science of medicine before this time? What had happened to the Hippocratic corpus of observation which was the beginning of medical science as we know it? Such scientific contributions as Hippocrates and his school made consisted of observations of the patterns of symptoms and signs in hundreds of patients. Many of these case-histories have come down to us. From these one can see the Hippocratic doctors working out the prognosis of the patient. Prognosis consists of forecasting the future of the patient. The treatment given by the Hippocratic doctors was of the simplest. It consisted mostly of a regime of diet, physiotherapy and a few drugs. It was full of commonsense, and allowed for the fact that treatment might harm as well as help a patient. Thus it was not dramatic and did not appeal to patients or doctors anything like as much as Galen's more sophisticated methods.

That any Greek medicine at all came down to us in the West through the darkness of the barbaric centuries following the fall of Rome is due to the work in the monasteries of the Christian Church. For it was the monks alone who had sufficient learning and compassion to apply the principles of Hippocratic or Galenic medicine to sick people.

The Renaissance presents us with the next great advance in medical science, which concerned human anatomy. The study of human anatomy for its own sake was introduced, for the first time since Galen, by the artist-scientist Leonardo da Vinci and the doctor Andreas Vesalius who exerted an enormous influence on posterity. However, such studies were mocked at by the practising doctors of the day who questioned what use they were in terms of treating sick patients. 'Little or none,' was the answer; so anatomy did not yet contribute much to the practice of medicine.

A similar reception was accorded to the work of William Harvey when he introduced the essential experimental method of physiological research. He thought out and performed a brilliant series of experiments from which he gained a comprehension of the nature of the action of the heart, and proved that the blood is propelled away from the heart in the arteries, returning back to the heart through the veins. In this way it circulates. But William Harvey's work on the heart was criticised by the age-old question, 'What use is this to medical practice?' Since the answer lay in the complete abandonment of Galenic ideas, it was not acceptable and it is strangely true that not only did Harvey's own practice fall after he had published his 'crack-brained' work on the heart in 1628, but his discovery had little or no effect on medical practice for more than a century afterwards.

In the eighteenth century a great anatomist, Morgagni, working in Italy, ended a life-long study of normal human anatomy by focusing his attention on the abnormal anatomy of disease (morbid anatomy). Morgagni made one most important further advance; he related the changes he found in diseased organs with the symptoms and signs which the patient had experienced in life. With this study he initiated a method of medical research which is still used today. Also, here at last was a method of discovery which could clearly be of use in medical practice. Doctors seized upon Morgagni's discoveries and methods with avidity for their value in diagnosing diseases in patients.

Diagnosis, which consists in obtaining a thorough knowledge of the nature and cause of a patient's disease, had now to be developed by fresh methods of examining the patient. Thus the method of percussion was introduced by the Viennese doctor Auenbrugger, who demonstrated that tapping the chest could show whether fluid or solid tissue lay beneath. Later Laennec introduced the stethoscope for listening to the sounds within the chest. Also in these early decades of the nineteenth century Dr Bright, working at Guy's Hospital in London, applied chemistry to the problems of kidney disease, so describing what we still call Bright's disease. All these new methods were beginning to make it possible to analyse the patient's disease further and to place it in a more scientific category according to its nature and causation.

But there was still a big gap between such advances in diagnosis and improvements in treatment. In fact the new knowledge of morbid anatomy and biochemical changes made treatment seem even more difficult, and there ensued a period of 'therapeutic nihilism' in which many of the best doctors found themselves unable to advise much treatment at all. The Galenic methods, it was agreed, must now be abandoned since they were founded on false principles. What was to replace them? If science could not supply the answer there remained only empiricism or nihilism. Empiricism implies treating by experience alone without the support of any theory. But, as Hippocrates warned, experience is deceptive; thus empiricism is perilous. What was there that a doctor could do for his patient in these circumstances? Many turned to Hippocrates for advice and found it in his discussion of epidemics where he wrote, 'The physician must have two special objects in view with regard to diseases, namely to do good or to do no harm.'[1] Thus the nineteenth-century doctor applied such theories as he trusted to the treatment of the patient; he used empirical treatments as his temperament and the circumstances demanded; and he consoled and comforted. With regard to consolation and comfort the doctor worked in close liaison with his colleague the clergyman. He studiously strove to do no harm; it was in this quest that he often approached the position of 'therapeutic nihilism'.

From about 1860 onwards medicine became rapidly more scientific. The sciences of physics and chemistry, of anatomy, physiology and pathology, not only grew on their own account, but were zealously incorporated into the practice of medicine. This process has continued even more rapidly in our own century, and through it knowledge of organic disease, that is disease of the bodily organs, has developed astoundingly. And sometimes by chance, sometimes as a result of logical research, very powerful methods of treating a number of organic diseases have been discovered. These have been mainly in three fields: in the treatment of many infections by antibiotics such as penicillin; in the treatment of endocrine disorders by hormones, e.g. diabetes by insulin; and in the surgical correction of mechanical faults, e.g. in the heart, blood-vessels and bones. It is false, however, to deduce from this that we are anywhere near 'the conquest of disease'. What we have done is to reduce enormously the impact of many diseases which used to kill the young, such as the acute infections. These are now being replaced by new, more chronic and elusive diseases; and more people are reaching the age when diseases of senescence take their toll. Many of these we cannot yet treat successfully. We have to realise that man must die; it is as natural for him to die as it is to be born. And when he dies, he generally dies of disease.

During the last century therefore we have been dramatically successful in applying the principles of physics and chemistry, through anatomy, physiology and pathology, to the diagnosis and treatment of disease. So successful indeed that we have run into the danger of treating the patient's physical and chemical state rather than the human being. This tendency has been counteracted by a movement that may perhaps be ascribed to such men as Charcot, Janet and Freud whereby emphasis has been placed on the patient's psyche, both conscious and unconscious. As these concepts have developed the psychoanalyst and the psychiatrist have taken over the part that the clergyman played a century ago. In doing so they have restored attention to the fact that a doctor is treating the whole person and not just a conglomeration of organs with their physico-chemical errors. They have also for the first time in medical history squeezed religion out of medical treatment.

Medicine and Society
Man is a social animal, and in touching on the treatment of emotional states we shift our attention from the patient ex-

clusively as an individual to the social sources of the patient's emotions. Centred in infancy on himself, these gradually spread through personal contact with parents, family and school, out into the world at large, into adult social life. Each stage of development involves both physical and mental growth, and adjustments which may provide stresses capable of upsetting the delicate harmonious interplay between the physical and emotional facets of the individual. Illness may arise from such discords, and the fact that in this twentieth century the physical and social environment of man changes with unprecedented rapidity, brings unprecedented emotional stresses demanding adjustments.

Rapid social changes such as we now experience emphasise the emotional sacrifice every individual has to make in order to adapt himself to the changing conventions and rules of his social milieu. They constitute a big price to be paid for our civilisation. Such sacrifices are too great for some, and they break down, expressing their distress in the form of mental disease.

The moulding forces of society, however, are by no means predominantly pathogenic. On the contrary, from the very earliest days of social organisation there has been a preventive and hygienic aspect of medicine which expresses the direct concern of those in power for the health of the people. This aspect of medicine is relatively impersonal; it has therefore often lain outside the province of practising doctors. It has involved the law-givers. This is evident, for example, in the Mosaic Code as expressed in the books of Leviticus and Deuteronomy. Here rules of hygiene and dietetic laws were laid down, some of which were of undoubted prophylactic value with regard to infectious diseases, while others encouraged habits of healthy living.

The first physician to give systematic attention to this hygienic aspect of medicine was the great Greek Hippocrates. This he considers in a long work entitled 'Airs, Waters and Places'. It is clear from this title that we have here a work in which the habits of society are taken into medical account. It has been described as 'the oldest exposition which we possess of the opinions entertained by an original and enlightened mind on many important questions connected with Public Hygiene and Political Economy'.[2]

In ancient Egypt, Greece and Rome admirable examples of public hygiene were to be found, though these were usually confined to the houses of the rich, rarely extending systematically over the countryside. In cities like Rome and Pompeii the whole population benefited. After the fall of Rome however hygiene became a forgotten and despised practice. Whilst the monks and nuns of the Christian Church came to the rescue in the practice of medicine on sick individuals, the same cannot be said with regard to their influence on hygiene. In so far as the medieval Christian attitude looked upon life on earth as a vale of tears and concentrated on life after death, it was not conductive to the development of hygienic advances. Indeed during the Middle Ages, and even as late as the nineteenth century, the Christian concept of the body as a merely temporary dwelling place for the soul, one in which there should be acceptance of suffering, led to the neglect of the prevention of that suffering by hygiene and public health.

Thus little attention was given to the health of the community in the planning of the medieval European towns and cities. These grew up as conglomerations of villages, and the inhabitants retained their old habits of throwing their solid or liquid refuse into the streets. Human excreta soiled the roads and paths, and the only attempt to clear it up were made by the night soil men who took it out for use on the land as manure. As the cities grew their sanitation became worse; for as buildings became more congested open spaces shrank. Thus it was at the end of the Middle Ages that city sanitation reached its worst plight.

Attempts to cope with the insanitary nuisance began in 1388 in England when Parliament passed an Act forbidding the throwing of filth and garbage into ditches and rivers. The planning of cities to meet the demands of health, hygiene and aesthetic harmony was envisaged by such men as Leon Battista Alberti in the fifteenth century who devoted a chapter of his work on architecture to drains and sewers, a subject further developed by Leonardo da Vinci in his designs for ideal towns of about 30,000 inhabitants with standardised prefabricated homes for the workers.

Disease is inevitably a social phenomenon since it not only harms the sick person but involves those in contact with him. In the case of infectious disease the sick man is a direct menace to the health of his fellow men. This was recognised in the Mosaic Code; and the regulations of Leviticus were put into practice on a large scale in Europe in the Middle Ages to combat leprosy and plague. It was appreciated that plague was brought in from the East chiefly by ships entering European ports. Thus in 1377 the city council of Ragusa ordered that travellers should not be admitted until they had spent one month of isolation on the island of Mercana. Venice soon followed suit, extending the period to forty days. Thus originated the practice called 'quarantine' so vital in the control of epidemic diseases even today. It was hoped thereby to prevent a repetition of the Black Death of 1345 which eliminated almost half the population of Europe.

These concepts of health maintenance, it will be noticed, did not emanate from the physicians, but came from enlightened non-medical individuals or legislative bodies such as the English parliament or the city council of Ragusa. Increasingly as time went on the physicians were called in to advise regarding such legislation. Sometimes they drew attention to special health dangers, as when William Harvey refers to London as 'a city whose great characteristic is an immense concourse of men and animals; where ditches abound and filth and offal lie scattered about, to say nothing of the smoke engendered by the general use of sulphureous coal as fuel whereby the air is at all times rendered heavy. . . . Such an atmosphere could not have been found otherwise than insalubrious.'[3] John Evelyn's *'Fumifugium, or The Smoake of London Dissipated,*[4] published a few years later (1661) sounds almost like an administrator's answer to Harvey's expostulation.

Gradually it came to be appreciated that the administration of public health was an important function of governments. Laws and ordinances concerning public health were more frequently enacted and enforced. But their effectiveness was severely limited by the insufficiency of medical science on the one hand, and the ruler's ignorance of medicine on the other. Despotic rule, common on the European continent in the seventeenth and eighteenth centuries, had an administrative advantage here. And Johann Peter Frank, a physician who was fully aware of the benefits of public hygiene, became adviser on this subject to several despotic monarchs, thus putting into practice his sound theory that rulers must be taught to keep their subjects healthy. Good health laws, in Frank's view, should be enforced by medical police.

Not until the second half of the nineteenth century did sanitary reform and public health organisation find their way into more liberally governed Britain. Leaders of this movement were disciples of that utilitarian philosopher, Jeremy Bentham, who spent his life devising schemes to 'promote the greatest happiness of the greatest number'. In 1821 Southwood Smith, a Nonconformist minister who had qualified as a doctor, settled in London and began to help Bentham to draw up a code for a ministry of health. This was in fact in anticipation of our National Health Service. Smith lived in the East End of London, and knew from first hand experience the conditions in the tenements of Shoreditch and Bethnal Green. He enlisted the help of a young lawyer, Chadwick, who was later made secretary of the Poor Law Commission which was set up under the Poor Law Act of 1834, and appointed to report officially on the sanitary conditions of the people. As a result the organisation of our Public Health system was undertaken by Sir John Simon, the first Medical Officer to the City of London, and Chief Medical Officer to the Privy Council. It was he who prepared the great Public Health Act of 1875 which brought a dramatic revolution of living conditions in Great Britain, providing that basic pattern of public hygiene which so many of us accept and take for granted today.

A similar story of the combined efforts of medical and non-medical citizens could be told in relation to the development of hospitals. These buildings represent a very old social ideal as centres of care for the sick and poor. At first this was part of the priest-physicians' task in the temples of ancient Egypt and the Aesculapian temples of Greece. The example was carried over into Roman times. In Rome itself the remnant of an Aesculapian temple still stands in the middle of the Tiber. In A.D. 360 St Basil incorporated hospitals into the Christian outlook on disease, building in Caesarea a whole hospital city. Later Moslem hospitals were founded all over the Arab world, one at Damascus being built as early as A.D. 707 by the Caliph. The Al-Mansur Hospital in Cairo boasted courtyards with fountains, diet kitchens, lecture rooms and a library, besides wards for special diseases. Europe's oldest general hospital was the Hotel Dieu in Paris with 1200 beds, founded in A.D. 660 by Landry, Bishop of Paris. It is still very active today. Pope Innocent III's example of building a Hospital of the Holy Ghost in Rome in the thirteenth century spread throughout Europe. Two of our London hospitals owe their origin to monks, St Bartholomew's to Rahere in A.D. 1123, and St Thomas's to Peter, Bishop of Winchester, in 1215. From these examples the dominant part played by the Christian and Moslem religions in this aspect of the care of the sick is very evident.

In England with the dissolution of the monasteries by Henry VIII the monastic hospitals disappeared, and their population of sick and beggared people was let loose to roam the countryside. It took two centuries before secular charity assumed the task previously borne by monastic charity. The Westminster Hospital, at first called an infirmary, was founded in 1719, and a few years later Thomas Guy, a wealthy bookseller, founded the hospital which bears his name. Others, such as the St George's and Middlesex Hospitals, soon followed. Though doctors played their part in planning, advising and working for these hospitals, secular Christian charity was their underlying motive force. But with the advances in medicine involving a vastly increased expense in the treatment of patients, private charity has been overstrained and the State has taken over the burden of building and maintaining hospitals. This has meant an ever-increasing responsibility being laid upon the patients and their representatives, i.e. the public, for the conditions under which medicine is practised.

Medical Ethics

It will be noticed that whether medicine is practised as a personal art between doctor and patient, or in an impersonal form as public health, it expresses an outlook which can be described as the medical ethic. This holds true whether the medical activity is performed by doctor or layman. Medical ethics constitutes perhaps the strongest and most constant thread of medicine, which is woven throughout the whole of human history, and binds its personal and public aspects together. Once more we find evidence of its origins in ancient times, as far back as the code of Hammurabi (about 1950 B.C.) where doctors' fees and the penalties for faulty treatment were regulated; for example, if an operation on an eye resulted in its loss the doctor's hands were cut off. Crude though this is, it is ethics.

With Hippocrates there appeared a less vindictive ethical code, so much more akin to our own views that we preserve many of its ideals today. The Hippocratic Oath however concerns itself almost entirely with the doctor's relationship to the patient. It ignores the reality of the patient's code of behaviour in relation to the doctor, or to fellow patients, either in the individual or collective sense. In this very brief survey of the role of medicine in history it is evident (though but rarely recognised) that the doctor constitutes somewhat less than half the story. There has been for too long a curious blindness to the other half of the theme, the healthy and unhealthy members of the public for whom medicine, therapeutic or preventive, is practised. Their knowledge and ethics are of as great importance as the knowledge and ethics of the doctor for the successful integration of medical practice in a community.

The term 'medical ethics' would in fact be more just and true if it were used to express the motive of efforts made by all of us as members of society to preserve or restore the mental or physical health of others. Expressed thus, the significance of medical ethics would become clearer to the general public, to the politician, lawyer, theologian and industrialist, all of whom besides the doctor are in fact working for their own aspect of this ideal. The preservation and restoration of health (though given so little thought by the healthy) are basic requirements of us all. Far from their being automatic rights we can at best obtain them over a limited span of life, and our objective is to enlarge and enrich that span.

It is often said that the ethics of medicine is exceptional in society, that the ethical demands made by the Hippocratic Oath exceed the capacities of those working in occupations other than medicine. If this is so the future outlook for our society is indeed gloomy, but the very existence of medical ethics throughout history, and the large part played in that story by non-medical men contradicts so sad a diagnosis.

In this section I have tried to show that one of the most noticeable and encouraging features of medical evolution during the last two hundred years has been the ever-increasing part played by the laymen who provide the para-medical services. And when one considers today how small a percentage of those who work in any ordinary general hospital is composed of qualified doctors, one realises what a large part of medical care is in fact provided by non-medical persons motivated at least in part by the influence of medical ethics. Indeed there is evidence that this influence already extends widely into our present-day society. I have heard it expressed by industrial scientists employed in researches with anything but medical end-products; and it sometimes finds expression in the unexpected actions of the most cynical of our citizens.

Medicine's Future Role

History has shown medicine running for centuries like an isolated thread through the texture of our society. Recently this thread has broadened, though we are largely unaware of the change. The further growth of a medical ethic combined with an increase of basic medical knowledge is gradually occurring. It needs a new vigorous thrust. Further expansion of this knowledge with its ethic into the worlds of the industrialist, the legislator, and even the theologian, would bring a logical and acceptable basis for the enrichment of all their activities, not to mention an improvement in the health of our very sick human society.

Is it enough, we may ask ourselves, for medicine to concern itself only with the prevention and treatment of disease? Although practising doctors would be inclined to answer, unhesitatingly, yes; and to add that with the recent pace of medical advance the task of preventing and treating bodily and mental ailments is not only enough but is already too much to cope with, yet they have still more to offer.

History has revealed that the ethic of medicine, however imperfectly practised by doctors, today stands almost alone in its acceptance by our materialistic society as a practical form of higher moral living. This is because it is based on knowledge and values arising from the basic events of human experience, birth and death, sickness and health. Thus medicine is essentially humanist in its outlook; all human experience, joys and sorrows, at higher as well as lower levels, are within its province. Without medical knowledge these events cannot possibly be understood nor evaluated. With medical knowledge there opens up a possible path of integration of personal experience, not to be derived from the purer, more defined sciences. For those fragmented abstractions of reality which we call 'pure' sciences cannot concern themselves with the evaluation even of the very virtues which their practice represents. Medicine, since it includes many of them in its purview, can and must see them, as well as itself, in the context of human values.

For some men the marvels of human achievement and potential are enough to absorb all their religious energy; for them perfection of human living is their religious ritual. Amongst them are many scientists and doctors. For many others however, this is not enough, for they feel the existence of greater forces.

It is historically true that in those parts of the world peopled by Europeans the ethic of medicine has grown from its ancient Greek nature through Christian nurture to its present form. Many doctors have found their ethic of medicine thus compounded, and along this path have reached their comprehension of experiences described by such words as 'God', 'holy', or 'divine' which play no part in an atheist or humanist vocabulary. Since it is true, however, that our

European ethical standards have in history been built upon Christian foundations medicine and its ethic are now in a position to open up a path to a re-doctrinated, re-formed Christianity potent to find a way to revive men's fading experience of faith, and to resensitise the awareness of the feelings of mystery and awe so dulled in our age. Thus through medicine could be created a renewed, revitalised form of Christianity. Similar problems confront the adaptation of other religious forms such as those of the Moslems and Hindus. Vastly different though their particular adjustments may be, they too need to pass through the common path of medicine and its ethics to emerge adapted to modern needs.

It could be the future of medicine to restore those creative fields of religious emotions so sadly and unnecessarily depressed by the fruits of the tree of knowledge. It could be the future of medicine to restore to men made so dangerously ataxic by their lost sense of religion the new healthy experience of coordinated power and inspired action.

REFERENCES

(1) HIPPOCRATES: 'Epidemics', Book 1, Section 2. Quoted from F. ADAMS: 'The Genuine Works of Hippocrates' (The Sydenham Society, 1849), Volume 1, p. 360.

(2) F. ADAMS: 'The Genuine Works of Hippocrates' (The Sydenham Society, 1849), Volume 1, p. 183.

(3) W. HARVEY: 'Anatomical Examination of the Body of Thomas Parr' Quoted from R. WILLIS: 'The Works of William Harvey' (The Sydenham Society, 1847), p. 591.

(4) J. EVELYN: 'Fumifugium or the Inconvenience of the Aer and Smoake of London Dissipated, together with some Remedies humbly proposed by John Evelyn Esq. to His Sacred Majestie and to the Parliament now Assembled' (W. Godbid, 1661).

2

THE HEALTH OF THE NATION

C. METCALFE BROWN, M.D., CH.B., D.P.H.

Dr Metcalfe Brown was formerly Medical Officer of Health of the City of Manchester and Lecturer in Preventive Medicine at Manchester University.

The nation's health is the health of its individual citizens collectively. The health of each national depends on heredity; on ante-natal health; on the environment, which includes home and the surroundings of the home, school and college, work-place, streets, and transport facilities; on nutrition; and on the standard and ready accessibility of medical care and treatment.

Man has a tremendous capacity of withstanding, overcoming or adapting himself to hardship and difficulties. Indeed, meeting the challenges of life provides for most but not all people the opportunity of fitting themselves for further improvement and progress, not only in health but in relation to human activities generally.

HEREDITY

The physical characteristics of our ancestors recur to some extent in ourselves. Auburn hair or brown eyes may be reproduced in some of the descendants 'unto the third and fourth generation' and many more. Similarly a capacity for resisting or failing to resist disease may sometimes be transmitted to offspring and if transmitted may follow a particular pattern. Haemophilia, an inherited blood condition, is restricted to male children but is transmitted by females of the affected family. Generally, normal parents have normal children and abnormal parents may or may not have abnormal children. Fortunately, what is known as mutation can occur; the genes that carry our heredity are not unalterable, and the tendency to abnormal characteristics in a family often disappears in the course of the successive generations. It has been said that because of mutation, hereditary defects in some may be the price of progress in the development of the race – the greater the mutation rate and hence the rate of change, the greater the incidence of defects. If this unhappy thought be true it means that the unfortunate few suffer for the greater benefit of the many.

INJURY OR INFECTION AT OR BEFORE BIRTH

Injury at birth may cause irreversible changes in a child resulting in a lifelong handicap, such as a paralysed limb or mental subnormality. Congenital defects may occur as a result of virus infection of the mother, for example from German measles in the second month of pregnancy, while epilepsy is a disorder of the nervous system which may be hereditary or the result of ante-natal infection or of injury at birth or injury at any time.

THE INFLUENCE OF ENVIRONMENT

Environment continues to be a major factor in relation to the public health. A recent book with American sponsors carries the title 'Health is a Community Affair', and indeed it is, but this is no new concept. In 1847 the Council of the Borough of Liverpool appointed a Medical Officer of Health 'to inspect and report periodically on the sanitary condition of the said borough, to ascertain the existence of diseases ... to point out the most efficacious modes for checking or preventing the spread of diseases and also to point out the most efficient means of ventilation of public edifices.' All honour to Liverpool as pioneers in preventive medicine in putting into practice the admonition of Moryson in 1617 to 'Appoint Chiefe men to the office of providing for the public health, calling the place where they meete, the Office of Health'.

From this we gather that health was deemed to depend largely on physical conditions and on the control of infectious diseases, and how right this was in bygone centuries. Even in modern times these factors are still important with some shift of emphasis as a result of greater knowledge, increased population and the advent of new health hazards.

Housing

A good house is the structural element of a good home – the place where a family begins, where children are born and reared, where husband and wife in marital harmony provide the background for happiness, comfort and mutual support – a soundly based part of society influencing and being influenced by other components of the community. It follows that housing is of very great importance. There is much good housing in Britain particularly in the south and in the areas on the fringe of the great conurbations but there is much bad housing nearer the centre of the conurbations. The worst areas in relation to quantity and bad quality of houses are London's East End, Glasgow, Liverpool, Manchester and Birmingham. Some bad housing is found in practically every village and town except in New Towns and the recently developed areas. Glasgow, in spite of strenuous efforts in providing new houses, still has very many old blocks of tenements with common entries, stone stairs to the upper apartments, and water closets adjacent to these stairs, serving two, three or four families. Leeds and other urban areas in the West Riding of Yorkshire still have the huge problem of replacing the remaining back to back houses, and Manchester with thousands of rows of unfit terraced houses still faces in spite of vast slum clearance a formidable task of more clearance and a vast programme of house construction.

The principal defects in bad housing are dampness, poor ventilation, poor lighting, inadequate sanitation and disrepair. These conditions cause or exacerbate disease in the occupants, principally the young and the very old; acute respiratory disease, gastro-intestinal disease and chronic bronchitis are rife. It is impossible to estimate the extent of the adverse psychological effects of bad housing on the tenants but it must be considerable.

In some industrial areas, smoke pollution has been tackled with vigour and there has been such a reduction of smoke from industrial undertakings that the 50% share of the responsibility of industry for smoke pollution has fallen to about 20%, the remainder being caused by dwelling houses. The nearer the chimney tops are to the ground the greater is the fall of soot locally and the pollution of the air around houses which are old and congested is greater than elsewhere. Smoke is not the only problem – other pollutants, some invisible, are believed to be at least as noxious; amongst other effects they cause or exacerbate bronchitis, acute and chronic, a common scourge of those who have to live in this kind of environment.

Smoke control has improved many residential areas from the point of view of health, but progress has slowed down partly for economic reasons and partly because old slums burning raw bituminous coal are still in existence in industrial areas and not worth converting for burning smokeless fuel.

School and Work

The improvement of school buildings and the increasing recognition of the need for adequate playing fields is a welcome and much needed development in providing a satisfactory environment for the children. There are however many unsatisfactory schools both in urban and rural areas and unfortunately and unfairly these schools are often found in the same area as the bad dwelling houses from which their pupils are drawn. The pupils therefore have the worst of both worlds; they live and sleep in slums and have to attend slum schools. In many of these slum schools the standard of education is good but would be better were it not for the overcrowding. Education includes health education and both teachers and school health visitors do much to inculcate habits of hygiene which will help the children to know the need for and how to achieve better standards of health.

Occupational health is being pursued with vigour as a result of the Factory Acts and the Offices, Shops and Railway Premises Act of 1963 which enforce reasonable standards in relation to work environment. The prevention of industrial diseases and the medical care of victims of accidents are well provided for by most of the larger industrial groups. The speed with which these facilities spread throughout industry will determine the speed with which health standards are raised for employees.

Transport

The continued growth of the large industrial and commercial areas of this country and the creation of residential areas at increasing distances from the centre means that more people are travelling greater distances to their places of employment. The hazards here are road accidents, increased risk of infection in overcrowded trains and buses, and increased pollution of the atmosphere by the invisible and at times all too visible products of combustion of the petrol and the Diesel engines of road vehicles. As to the first, road accidents will tend to increase as road traffic increases, causing more deaths and permanent injury to drivers and passengers. The increasing use of safety measures and devices does however help to reduce the effects of the progressive incidence of road accidents in recent years. As to the second, the travelling public appears to develop immunities to the infections of other people in crowded places, except in times of epidemic, for example influenza. As to the third, the air pollution from motor traffic is added to that from heating appliances, coal fires and oil burners, and while towns are losing their visible smoke there is no corresponding decrease of invisible pollutants.

NUTRITION

The rising prosperity of the nation and the increasing understanding of the need for adequate and well-balanced diets for children and adults alike has done much to improve the health of the people of Britain. Economic prosperity is a first condition of improved nutrition because poverty makes it impossible to buy an adequate amount of first class foods. There is still a good deal of ignorance about what foods these are and how to prepare and cook them. Proteins provide the materials required for growth and the replacement of worn-out body tissues. They, like carbohydrates and fats, provide the sources of physical energy. They tend to be the most expensive foods and in consequence they are not available in sufficient quantities to families who are poor in money or poor in understanding, or both. Fats are essential for a balanced diet. Too little means loss of energy, while too much may cause arterial disease, including coronary disease, in people who are too well fed and too little exercised.

Carbohydrates, the cheapest form of food, provide energy and in excess are converted into fat after digestion. Children with their enormous output of energy need plenty of carbohydrates as well as protein, but this can be overdone causing the familiar picture of obesity in children. There is little doubt that far too many children and some adults consume much more cane sugar than is good for their health – too many sweets in the case of children.

Food in Britain is adequate in amount, but carbohydrate consumption, particularly in the form of refined sugar, should be curbed. In adults, too much alcohol is harmful to health, but small amounts relax tension and used in moderation socially induce a capacity to mix well with other people to mutual advantage.

Vitamins, of which there are many, are essential for the maintenance of good health. These occur in sufficient quantity in a good varied diet. Deficiency of some of them may result in serious affections.

MEDICAL CARE AND TREATMENT

The health services in Britain are divided into three parts, (a) hospital and consultant service, (b) general medical, dental and pharmaceutical services, and (c) local health authority services.

The Hospital Service

The hospital service is too well known to require a detailed description here. Admission to hospital under the National Health Service Act is secured for the patient by his general practitioner. The consultant and other hospital doctors provide whatever care, diagnosis and treatment may be required and the costs are met by the appropriate Regional Hospital Board and not by the patient. Arrangements however do exist for the treatment of private patients at appropriate charges. The work of the hospitals has expanded greatly in the twenty-three years of the present hospital scheme and has contributed greatly to the attainment of the high standard of health of this country.

General Practitioner and Dental Services

The general practitioner is essentially the family doctor in charge of all aspects of the health of the individual, or as often as not, of all the individuals in one family. This latter is important because the health of the patient is related to and influenced by the health background of the other members of the family to which he belongs. The general practitioner examines, advises and treats any patient on his list who requires his services, and the patient who co-operates with him in a good doctor-patient relationship has much to be thankful for and will benefit in health accordingly.

Local Health Authority Services

The primary duty of consultants and general practitioners in caring for their patients is to ensure that the interests of their patients are paramount. But there is also another interest which must be safeguarded – the health of the community. This means preventive medicine, which is provided for mainly by local authorities.

Thirty years ago diphtheria and virulent scarlet fever were rife, but these infectious diseases have now been subdued. However there must still be vigilance in relation to these diseases, as well as typhoid fever and poliomyelitis, while in the young, measles and whooping cough require the closest attention. The epidemiology of infectious diseases is dealt with by the Local Health Authority through the Medical Officer of Health; he has also many other duties.

Health Centres

Local Health Authorities are empowered to provide health centres and many do so, but the provision is far short of the need. A comprehensive service, and this is the ideal kind, provides accommodation for general practitioners, consulting rooms, examination rooms or cubicles, waiting rooms and accommodation for other staff concerned in the work of the centre – dental surgeons, health visitors, midwives, nurses, receptionists and clerical staff. Here a number of doctors work together, not necessarily in partnership, but closely associated; they provide a twenty-four-hour service for the patients on the doctors' lists and have facilities for consulting together on medical matters generally, and if necessary about individual patients when a joint opinion is thought likely to help the patient. Here the preventive work of the Local Authority will be carried out in association with the medical staff of the centre. Here also will the necessary immunizations of children be arranged, the records perhaps being kept by computors, and reminders for attendances sent to the parents at particular dates calculated and recorded by the computors. The commoner immunizations are against smallpox, diphtheria, tetanus, whooping cough, measles, and poliomyelitis, but other immunizations are given as required to young and old. As a result, millions of children in Britain have been protected against these diseases and thousands of deaths have been prevented. It is little wonder that infant mortality is about one tenth of what it was at the turn of the century.

Health Visiting

In every town and county there is a team of health visitors – trained nurses with special qualifications for social work – who attend the centres or clinics for mothers and babies and who visit their homes to advise and help all members of each family about their health, if this is acceptable to them. The health visitor also visits the schools and advises the teaching staffs on health matters affecting the schoolchildren and inspects the children themselves, keeping a watchful eye on their physical and mental welfare. The School Medical Officers carry out medical examination of the children at school at intervals and also as required in special cases drawn to their attention by the teachers or the health visitors. Children with minor ailments are sent to school clinics or health centres for treatment and there are clinics for special work staffed by doctors, for example, for ophthalmic treatment and for rheumatism and cardiac ailments.

Home Nursing

District nurses provide an efficient service of nursing care, visiting the homes of patients who do not require hospital service but need frequent visits from trained nurses to attend to their needs. This is a most valuable service much appreciated in particular by the old and infirm and the bedridden and their relatives.

Mental Health Service

Fifty years ago mental patients were locked up in asylums, as they were called, usually situated far away in the country in pleasant but often isolated surroundings, and there most of them stayed until they died, their original mental condition having deteriorated further as a result of well-meaning but wrong incarceration. Today the permanent population of the mental hospitals is much less than it used to be. Most patients with mental illness stay there for a relatively short period and return home cured, or with their condition alleviated, or on trial at home with the right to return to hospital if they need further treatment. Very many patients never need to go to hospital; they are treated by their own doctors and supervised in their own interests by the mental health visitors who also have the care of patients who have returned from hospital. Thus we now have an enlightened and helpful system of mental health care. Mental difficulties are regarded as illness and given appropriate treatment just as physical ailments are.

SIGNPOSTS OF PROGRESS

Infant Mortality Rate

This is one of the most sensitive indices for measuring progress in health matters, particularly in relation to environment. The rate is expressed for England and Wales as the

28

number of deaths in children dying under one year of age per 1000 live births in the area concerned.

Infant Mortality Rate – England and Wales

Year	Rate
1891	149
1901	151
1911	130
1921	83
1931	66
1941	60
1951	30
1961	21
1968	18

In Dundee, Scotland, the rate in 1891 was 203 and in 1900 it was 199, so that of every five children born in that city at that time, one died before reaching the age of one year. Now the figure is only about one in fifty.

Maternal Mortality Rate

This is the number of mothers who die from causes associated with childbirth per 1000 total births.

Year	Rate
1935	4.33
1941	2.80
1951	0.76
1961	0.33
1968	0.24

The advent of antibiotic treatment is no doubt the most important factor influencing this favourable result, and this too is a factor in the reduction of the infant mortality rate.

Infectious Diseases

The death rate from tuberculosis is now approximately 1.30 per cent of that of 100 years ago; antibiotic therapy is an important but not the only factor here. Vaccination has eliminated smallpox in the United Kingdom, except for sporadic outbreaks. Poliomyelitis is practically eliminated in the United Kingdom because of systematic immunization with attenuated live polio virus. Diphtheria is now very rare indeed as a result of immunization.

Cigarette Smoking

The Chief Medical Officer in his annual report for 1967 on the state of the public health, wrote: 'Death and disability due to smoking cigarettes continued to increase during the year 1967.' The annual report for 1966 recorded that 'the number of deaths which can be fairly attributed to smoking – from cancer, bronchitis and heart disease – must have exceeded 50,000' and went on to say that this was an underestimate.

Venereal Disease

The Chief Medical Officer's report for 1967 stated that: 'Gonorrhoea has shown a further sharp increase in both men and women and the prospects for an early solution to this problem seem remote.'

Illegitimate Births

The following table shows the progressive increase in the number of illegitimate births per 1,000 unmarried women aged 15-44 in the years indicated.

Year	Number
1950	10.2
1955	10.3
1960	15.1
1964	19.9
1965	21.2
1966	21.5
1967	22.6

They now represent more than 16.0 per cent of all births in the larger cities of this country. It is not surprising that the incidence of gonorrhoea also is increasing.

Here is clear evidence of a diminishing standard of

morality and of a very low level of responsibility. The illegitimate child – more accurately the child of the illegitimate father and mother – is bereft at birth of all the advantages enjoyed by the children of normal well-founded families. Many such children do overcome their initial disadvantages and become good and useful citizens, but the dice are loaded against them.

The community that accepts an increasing number of illegitimate births does so at the peril of its future.

Alcohol and Drugs

The reasonable use of alcohol causes no damage to health but unreasonable use, too often and too much, is often disastrous for the alcoholic and for his family. Heavy drinking can and does lead to crime and matrimonial difficulties – and to serious mental disorders as well as physical deterioration.

In young people, drug addiction has reached alarming proportions with pitiable results for those who have been ensnared by this evil. Home Office statistics show that both cannabis offences and heroin addictions were at fairly stable, low levels in the mid-fifties; that both began to rise steeply about 1959; that both have now increased about twentyfold; and that neither shows any sign of levelling off. Ninetyfive per cent of the heroin addicts are under thirty-five. Even though addicts as such are relatively few – there were 2,782 known heroin addicts in 1968 – that number is far exceeded by that of young people who take drugs for 'kicks' but have not reached the parlous addicted state.

The remedy is better training and higher self-discipline. Adults who indulge too much in alcohol may well ask themselves whether they are setting a proper example to young people both in relation to alcohol and to drugs.

Suicide

In recent years, some 5,000 people annually in England and Wales have died by their own hand. Attempts at suicide far exceed the number of deaths – a sad indication of instability and unhappiness in a considerable number of people. Some lack of faith is obviously one factor; another is temporary or permanent mental ill health.

CONCLUSION

In matters of health there has been in Britain a recognition of the needs of people and this has caused investigation and a deeper knowledge of the problems involved and produced elaborate and extensive services to solve them. Many problems have been solved, but many have not, and newer ones have appeared. A long time ago Sir William Osler, a distinguished physician and professor of medicine, wrote about tuberculosis, 'Much has been done, much remains to do,' and that sentiment may well be echoed about what are now much more serious problems than tuberculosis, affecting both personal and public health. The health of the nation has improved enormously since the end of the Second World War, and the costs of achieving this for hospital and general medical services in England, Scotland and Wales is approximately one thousand million pounds per annum, which may well be thought much money well spent. This is good reason for satisfaction but there is no room for complacency. There are clear signposts of progress and also of regression. Increasing cigarette smoking causes serious ill-health and many deaths – sure evidence that there is a lack of self-discipline in the community in relation to health, as well as ignorance, which in view of much propaganda and admonition is no longer a defence nor a reasonable excuse.

The prospects of an early answer to the further sharp increase of the incidence of gonorrhoea are indeed remote. This increase is an indication of increasing sexual promiscuity, and the progressive increase in the number of illegitimate births is a sure sign of some deterioration in moral values in a nation which enjoys one of the best health services in the world.

Most of us enjoy good physical and mental health, but what of spiritual health? 'We have left undone those things which we ought to have done; And we have done those things which we ought not to have done; And there is no health in us.' If this be true the remedy for the nation is in the hands of the nation.

Britain and some other countries have led the world in many respects in the cause of humanitarianism and civilization. Many other nations are now emerging from a state of backwardness and they must be conscious that we ourselves are failing to show a good example. It is essential that we should accept individually and collectively the responsibility of demonstrating how well a healthy nation can live and above all why it does so.

3

SOME ETHICAL PROBLEMS FACING MEDICINE

PROFESSOR FRANCIS E. CAMPS
M.D., F.R.C.P., F.C.PATH., D.T.M. & H., D.M.J.

Professor Camps is Director of Department of Forensic Medicine at The London Hospital Medical College, and is the Home Office Pathologist.

Advances in science and medicine during the last few years have outstepped the moral and ethical conceptions of the past. In some cases this situation demands a 'new look' or rethinking as to how the present position can or should be reconciled with hitherto accepted and acceptable ideas. Perhaps the most challenging issues are those concerned with life and death (including abortion and euthanasia), with human experimentation and with the use of drugs.

Death and Transplantation

Few ethical problems with which the community has been faced in the past have equalled those involved in defining death, for they are closely associated with the legislation of self destruction on the one hand and the philosophy of 'spare part' surgery on the other.

Fundamentally the issue concerns respect for the right of a normal human being to decide for himself whether he shall live or die and what shall be the fate of his body when he is dead or even during his life. The problem might be simpler if these decisions were always ones which he is capable of making or communicating himself. It was for example pointed out in the House of Lords debate on euthanasia in 1969 that a patient might change his mind at a stage when he is no longer able to tell the doctor what he wants.

Some Ethical Problems Facing Medicine

Whereas in the past death was regarded as an inevitable and respectable end of life, which once established left only the question of departure of the spirit and reverent disposal of a body accepted as expendable, the situation is now far more complicated. Previously, establishing death depended from a medical and legal point of view upon the clinical observation of a doctor to decide that breathing and circulation no longer persisted. Even then there was nevertheless some doubt that the observations might not be correct. This was demonstrated by requests for the radial artery to be severed lest premature burial took place. The possibility of *apparent* rather than *true* death was of course greater before sophisticated instrumental methods became available. Thus subjects with hypothermia may often in the past have been regarded as dead, but now an electrocardiograph must be taken to establish the diagnosis.

Moreover, reverence for death has not completely ceased to exist, for in the minds of many it is the rational end of life and as such a supreme moment to be respected by those participating in and closely associated with the final situation. Yet even though the end is inevitable the medical profession may be confused by a natural sense of professional failure or guilt that a patient has 'slipped through its hands', and may display compensatory desire to prolong life by over-zealous treatment. This however can be dealt with by education, and the 'new approach' of maintaining a form of life at all costs has developed rather from the ability now available to restore 'life' by using mechanical methods to re-establish and maintain respiration and circulation. On such a basis 'death' need never occur so long as decomposition is absent, for a half-living state can be established and kept going after quite a considerable time and to such an extent that organs can be used for transplantation.

Nevertheless, if respiration and circulation are permitted to cease for a period and then artificially recommenced, the organs, although they may be viable and suitable for grafting into someone else who is living, are 'redundant' for the person who is effectively dead – except perhaps from an emotional point of view, which may well also be associated with religious belief. This conception has one grave difficulty insomuch as it may be suggested that the unknown quality, the 'spirit' or 'soul', might still be present. Those who do not believe in the hereafter, and hence in the soul, presumably would accept that death has occurred and that the organs are therefore available for other suitable uses. Even they, however, might on occasion pause to wonder whether the brain might still be 'alive' especially if they associate its functional activity with the 'power of thought'. Unfortunately, this is complicated by the fact that parts of the central nervous system are more sensitive to lack of blood supply than other tissues. Hence, there must be an assumption that 'brain death' occurs after an empirical period of cessation of blood supply during which other tissues continue to live. However, even if a specific time be accepted for this irreversible process (brain death) to occur but to leave the organs suitable for use, there still must be some people who find 'mutilation' of a human body unacceptable on religious or racial grounds.

Another aspect not always given proper consideration is the justification of a transplantation, when it may result in a protracted state of treatment with or without a terminal result. Certainly as things stand at present, the financial cost and the immediate results do not justify transplantation of hearts other than on the basis of the hope of future successes. So, too, unless success means substantially increasing the expectation of life for an individual, and not merely conferring a further short period of existence, it might well be thought that the benefit gained did not outweigh the other factors, although the case might be exciting and sensational when read in the newspapers. There must also be some doubts as to whether agreement by a close relative for a heart to be taken can be genuinely given under the emotional circumstances of sudden death.

It is moreover a somewhat paradoxical situation when on the one hand serious attempts are being made to reduce deaths from accidents, and on the other it is these very accidents that provide organs for transplantation. It is also paradoxical that more ill people should survive when the population explosion is causing anxiety.

The law of supply and demand has often caused problems in the past. As is well-known, there was a time when medical schools had difficulty in obtaining enough cadavers for their students to dissect. To meet the demand a nefarious traffic developed of snatching bodies from graves, and when even this proved insufficiently prolific some suppliers are said to have resorted to the surreptitious killing.

One wonders what may develop in future to meet the demand for spare parts, for as the demand grows there is certainly going to be an impasse. The fact that it is no longer illegal to commit suicide might well be used as an excuse. Whereas today a person may say, 'I want to commit suicide', tomorrow we may reach the stage where he says, 'I am going to commit suicide. I will come and do it in your hospital and you can have my organs.' If by then voluntary euthanasia has been legalised, what will happen? Shall we even get to the point where a surgeon wanting spare parts persuades a prospective suicide to 'volunteer'? In this permissive age the sanctity of the human body appears to become less, whilst justification for scientific advances by human experimentation becomes greater as opposition to and doubts about the validity of animal experiments increase. A recent appeal for more hearts on the grounds that some had died 'waiting' and others would also die if none became available is typical of the present trend and might well evoke the somewhat cynical but albeit realistic response of referring to the small number who have survived the operation.

Such a realistic, objective approach to transplants, according as it does with the rights of human beings to respect their religious and philosophical beliefs, must not be taken as opposition to the advancement of science or medicine. Moreover we must not be stampeded by the scientific demands of a minority, when the medical well-being of the majority is the greater need. Under similar circumstances in the past, the passage of time has brought its solution; in due course far more knowledge should be gained, especially with the help of a multi-disciplined approach including theological concepts, regarding the meaning and not merely the 'fact' of death. Tissue rejection, which is accepted as requiring much more study, may be construed as a deliberate attempt of nature to slow things down so as to allow more time for a clinical, theological and philosophical rather than a surgical approach to the treatment of the sickness of mankind. At the same time, advances in the transplantation of other tissues, such as kidneys and livers, which make less exacting demands on sources of material, may prove more rewarding for prolonged maintenance of life in younger people.

Human Experimentation

Other forms of human experimentation, such as clinical confirmatory tests to evaluate new drugs and new preventative measures, do not cause such grave misgivings. Nevertheless the very phrase 'human experimentation' arouses a certain feeling of revulsion, especially among those with memories of experiments carried out by the Nazis in concentration camps during the Second World War. Despite the present atmosphere of almost excessive permissiveness there has indeed been a hardening of opinion both within parts of the medical profession and amongst the public in relation to this topic, and it is consequently important to be clear about what is involved.

In one sense there must always be human experimentation if there is to be any progress at all. There must always be a first time that a new treatment or a new operation is performed on a human being. A new therapeutic drug, for example, is given an initial screening by animal experimentation, but once the drug is shown to have potential value there must come a time when it is administered to a human patient. Such a patient will be at risk from the point of view of side effects, but will stand to benefit if the drug produces positive results.

Another procedure which may be described as experimentation is that in which a diagnostic test is applied in order to decide what to do next. There are cases in which a dangerous procedure is essential, for instance an arteriogram to locate a cerebral aneurysm. It is important in such cases that enthusiasm for knowledge should not cloud the judgement, and that the procedures used should be genuinely necessary. The issue can usually be resolved by asking the simple question, 'Why?'

More controversial are procedures carried out to benefit others, rather than the patient himself or herself. These may undoubtedly have merits which can be argued even on ethical grounds. The degree of risk, which can vary from negligible to large, is obviously an important factor in making an assessment.

Before anything even remotely resembling experimentation is embarked on, certain basic principles must be accepted. Prime among these is obtaining the consent of the subject or responsible dependant. A. P. Beddard many years ago drew attention to the fact that the patients' bodies are their own property and not that of the medical profession, and this still holds good. Consent, moreover, can only be regarded as valid if the risks involved have been revealed.

The experimenter must also weigh degree of risk and the degree of benefit. The procedure if dangerous *must* be directed primarily towards the benefit of the subject. If on the other hand the risk is low, and benefits may accrue to others as a result of the advance in knowledge that occurs, then the doctor should evaluate the motivation in discussion with independent parties who have suitable experience. He must also be prepared to examine his own conscience; rules and the Law can deal with the blacks and whites, but the greys call for cross- and self-examination. With the rapidly growing opposition to animal experiments, it is important to resolve these issues, because the pressure to use human material to test new drugs and techniques is likely to increase.

Drugs

The third major problem in modern medicine is associated with the use of 'medicines'. At one public school many years ago there was a notice in the sick room which read as follows:

> Drugs cure the sick,
> but make the healthy ill

which brings us to the question of what is meant by a 'drug'. This is a purely scientific issue, depending on whether a substance changes either the physical or mental capacity of a person; thus one substance may lower the body temperature, and another may alter a person's approach to a problem. In the latter case, it may be directed to changing the attitude of an obsessional case and such an end may be desirable. Alternatively it may enable a person to avoid facing up to a problem whether it be personal or sociological. For example, a leader of state may be faced with a decision upon which the future of the world may depend; he can use his own judgement and experience unaided or he can ask his doctor for a tranquillising drug, but does this produce the right answer?

We all have before us the example of the Crucifixion – what happened there? Would it have so much impact if it was known that Christ had previously taken an analgesic and a tranquilliser? Of course not. The secret was the ability to face what life brought, not to avoid it.

Therapeutic drugs indeed bring us up against one of the problems of modern medicine, one which cannot be divorced from modern social science: shall the medical profession try in *all* cases to discover the many factors influencing a disease process, or avoid such a decision and treat the disease empirically by drugs alone? As a matter of fact it might well be worth while considering whether we desire a nation of people who avoid issues by taking drugs or who face up to those same issues and the relationships they involve. The one is an artificial, and the other a human approach.

It might be that in future we shall need to look at the matter from the point of view of reality *versus* artificiality. Tranquillising and stimulating drugs can be regarded as inducing artificial states, in which the true personality of the subject is suppressed. We may need to help our patients to rely on their power to think and make their own, un-drug-dictated decisions.

If I were writing a detective story about destroying the world, I would not bother about atom bombs and things like that. There are other ways which would be far more successful. Nowadays we have terrific powers to change

40

personality. For instance the well-known hallucinogen L.S.D. was produced partly with the idea of chemical warfare. The enemy would be having lovely dreams, and you would march in and take over. It is much easier than blowing everybody up. Even tranquillisers would go a long way—and what proportion of the population is on tranquillisers already?

Finally, there is the acute problem of drug dependence and addiction. This, involving as it does youth, is attributable in part to a combination of permissiveness and discontent. We do well to remember, however, that we have had certain socially acceptable drugs for centuries – alcohol, tobacco and we should even include coffee. These are all addictive in some subjects.

An alcoholic might be defined as a heavy drinker who has reached the stage when he cannot remember the next morning where he has left his car the night before. This is a danger sign, indicating that it is time to stop drinking or give up driving, neither of which is likely to occur without help. One alcoholic even drove all the way from Glasgow to London without remembering doing it. This sounds terrible, though the fact remains that he had no accident.

In the correct dosage alcohol produces gaiety and removes inhibitions, while an overdose can bring out aggressiveness. This is in the context of party excitement, but in the context of subsequent dispersal other things can happen, as can be seen from the condition of the gate-posts the following morning! Herein lies the paradox : one set of conditions leads to social success, another to over-confidence. This kind of thing is distinct from alcoholism though it can lead to it, and there are indeed two separate problems which require separate treatment. Social and habitual drinkers may need legal restraints to reduce accidents and other consequences, while the alcoholic should be regarded as suffering from a disease. Merely restricting supply may only aggravate the problem, as American experience with prohibition shows.

Alcoholism actually constitutes the largest of drug addiction problems, and they are all clinical and social icebergs – a quarter or less on the surface and the rest hidden and, I would go so far as say, administratively 'swept under the carpet'. From a social point of view they reduce productivity, cause immense family misery, and probably cut short the lives of some of the best brains.

The so-called 'soft' drugs, which include amphetamines, barbiturates and cannabis (also called marijuana, Indian hemp, or 'pot'), are not physiologically addictive, though one can become habituated to them by repeated consumption. That is to say, although there is a desire for the drug, there is little or no tendency to increase the dose, and dependence is psychic but not physical. The present wave of soft drug consumption is clearly epidemic, and should run its epidemiological course once publicity and antagonism to self-discipline have succumbed to inanition.

Meanwhile cannabis is brought into Britain, as flowers or resin, literally in tons. It must be recognised that it is a terrific incitement to people to pay for their holidays by bringing some back.

A pop singer recently attacked police attitudes to pop singers found in possession of cannabis, and came out with the superficial and much publicised claims that 'pot' is less harmful than alcohol, and that it does not lead on to harder drugs. On the former point she may well be right so far as the drug *per se* is concerned, but on the latter she seems to be unaware of the statistics presented by Professor W. D. M. Paton in 1968 to the British Association for the Advancement of Science. Obviously not all cannabis-takers progress to hard drugs, but Professor Paton calculates that 7–15% do go on to heroin, and that 88% of heroin-takers also take cannabis. It is in any case only commonsense to recognise that the cult of the one may lead to experimentation with the other. Pop stars have a duty not to encourage their fans down the slippery slope.

Addiction to hard drugs is a different problem from soft drug dependence, because although also epidemic and infectious in character, those who become infected are, as with alcoholism, very liable to relapse after cure. This is due in part at least to the inherent characteristics of hard drugs. In the present state of knowledge, the only real approach to treatment lies in 'support' from a psychological point of view. Legal restrictions on supply are at the best of very limited success, as has been seen elsewhere in the world. Treating drug addiction as an infectious disease we might isolate addicts to check the epidemic, but this would probably cause an outcry, so our hands are tied. Again, if it is a disease, we should not punish addicts, but the people who sell hard drugs illegally should be very heavily punished. It is no good fining them.

The whole drug problem undoubtedly arises partly from lack of 'something to believe in', and this is due to divorcement from *any* form of religious belief or conviction. A lot of rethinking and research is needed into the nature of addiction and dependence, and the future would seem to lie with a multi-disciplined approach, including religion.

Abortion

The problems however do not by any means finish here for there are those in which legislation conflicts with conceptions originally and still held by many of the community both on ethical and religious grounds. The latter may differ according to belief but this is no reason to ignore the feelings of a minority. As an example the new laws relating to abortion would have been acceptable to many had they merely legalised the right of a doctor to terminate pregnancy in order to save the life of the mother. A majority would also accept that it was justifiable to destroy the unborn child if continuation of the pregnancy was likely to cause mental breakdown or suicide, although study of the statistical evidence showed that suicide due to pregnancy was very rare and if it did occur was usually because of a pre-existing mental disease rather than the pregnancy itself.

However, the law was changed mainly on the basis that it was better to empty the uterus under proper surgical conditions legally than that the woman should go to a professional abortionist and risk her life, and also that if the members of the medical profession exercising their ethical standards did such an operation, it should be done without risk of prosecution. The latter argument was not completely realistic when examination of the records of the prosecution of registered medical practitioners showed that no conviction had ever taken place of any doctor who had followed the accepted code of procedure since the Bourne case. However, when the law was changed, although it made provision for certain safeguards, it equally opened the doors for legal misuse of what had previously been illegal practices inhibited by the possibility of legal proceedings.

Legislation is clearly of value to the community so long as it falls within the accepted conventional and ethical code but once it strays from within these boundaries then it defeats its own purposes and it was never intended that this legislation was for the purpose of encouraging promiscuous sexual intercourse and avoiding the conventional risks thereof. In fact this situation was adequately guarded by modern methods of contraception. Certainly it was not designed to assist those who had transgressed the moral and legal codes in other countries. Examination of changes in the law which superficially appear to offer advantages show that many have had unforseen consequences, a good example being the legislation of gambling.

Euthanasia and Venereal Disease

Recent new laws suggested in Parliament have included euthanasia and special legislation on venereal disease. The former issue will continue to be raised but it is difficult to see why the responsibility for taking a life should be acceptable when this was one of the main reasons for suspension of capital punishment. So too the control of the increasing incidence of venereal disease should be by restoration of proper standards of convention. Closely allied to many of the major social problems confronting the community is lack of self-discipline and without some standard of behaviour such as is an integral part of all religious beliefs this standard will continue to deteriorate.

4

MAN'S IMPACT ON THE ENVIRONMENT

H. A. C. MᶜKAY, M.A., D.SC.

Dr MᶜKay has been engaged in environmental studies in the course of his work at Harwell for the U.K. Atomic Energy Authority. The views expressed do not necessarily represent those of the Authority.

We live in a wonderful world – a world that provides air, water and food; clothing, shelter and fuel; the beauties of land, shore and sea; the endless fascination of the animal, plant and mineral kingdoms; rhythm, novelty and variety. Yet it is a world menaced by man swarming over its surface, and finding ever new and more drastic ways of exploiting it.

The Balance of Nature

Its natural state is normally one of balance. There are daily and seasonal changes, but over the years the climate and the populations of different species of flora and fauna in any given area remain roughly constant. This is because the basic physical factors, such as the amount of heat the earth receives from the sun, are fairly steady, and because the natural growth rates of animal and plant species are held in check by predators, by diseases, by food shortages, and so forth.

The processes that go on in the biosphere and produce this steady state are extraordinarily complex, and their study constitutes the science of ecology. Thus plants may provide food for insects, and may depend on them for pollination; birds may eat fruit and insects, and may use waste vegetation to make nests; carnivores catch and eat other animals; animal manure is broken down by micro-organisms and nourishes plants. Everywhere there is a complicated network of interactions, which combine to give a state of balance, and in every corner of the world the network is different.

Despite the complexities, the balance of nature is remarkably stable. It fluctuates from year to year, according to the weather and other factors, but only within certain limits, and if upset by an unusual event, such as a volcanic eruption, the balance is generally in due course re-established. This is because it is self-regulating. A hard winter may kill off numbers of birds, and this may give the flies a chance to multiply; but this in turn provides a superabundance of insect food for the next generation of birds, and so tends to restore the original state of affairs.

Nevertheless, over the millenia nature does change, as the fossil record shows. The balance is never permanent. Just as a person changes slowly throughout life, while maintaining an approximate energy and material balance between intake of air, water and food on the one hand, and activity and excretion on the other, so does nature slowly change.

Change occurs when the physical conditions of the environment change. The last ice age, for example, blotted out the existing natural balance over most of the northern hemisphere, and a new balance had to be established when the ice retreated. Change also occurs when a new biological factor is introduced. Thus myxomatosis almost eliminated rabbits in this country. This affected foxes, which turned to other animals for food, and hares, which increased in numbers when their chief competitors were removed. It also affected vegetation; grasses and shrubs were able to grow more freely, but other species were extinguished because the grasses cut off their light.

However, a rabbit-less balance has not been established because the rabbit is staging a come-back. A strain of myxomatosis-resistant rabbits has emerged. Resistance is believed to arise in a small proportion of the population as a result of chance variations (mutations), and since only the resistant rabbits survive and breed, virtually all rabbits today are of the new variety, and this can presumably fill essentially the same ecological niche as the old. Here we have natural selection at work, and as a result a species has successfully adapted itself to a new situation.

46

It is a most important feature of the picture that plant and animal species can change in this way. We have to deal not only with the balance between existing species, and changes in the balance in response to physical and biological changes in the environment, but also with variations in the bodily structure of the species themselves. Such variations arise spontaneously, and a variation in one species may favour a complementary adjustment in another species, so that a progressive series of changes may occur. The cumulative effect of a long series of variations may ultimately lead to the formation of new species.

The Impact of Man

Into the intricate balance of nature has come man. To start with he was part of it in much the same way as other living creatures. He fitted in, like them, to the ecology of his surroundings. Yet he was different, first because he fashioned and used tools and secondly because he had the gift of speech with all that that implies in storing and transmitting knowledge.

With these exceptional powers he began to have a unique impact on his environment. He sought consciously to modify it to his advantage, as when he started to farm, and later he created wholly new environments, as when he built towns and cities. We recognise man's special place when we draw a distinction between the man-made, or artificial, and the natural. Why otherwise should we, for example, regard a rabbit's or a bird's dwelling as natural, and man's as artificial?

Often man's efforts have created for a time a new balance, in which his activities are integrated with nature. In areas of settled farming, for example, the farms form part of the living pattern of the region. Micro-organisms in the soil, insect pollinators, birds that keep the insects in check, draught animals that also yield manure, all assist the farmer, and he, whether deliberately or not, helps to provide their livelihood. In some countries this state of affairs has persisted for centuries, and to city-bound, twentieth-century man it has a certain idyllic quality. Yet it cannot survive unchanged. Rising human populations and advances in farming technique alter the pattern continually and ever more rapidly.

Since the last ice age there has indeed never been a lasting equilibrium between mankind as a whole and the natural environment. If there were, the total human population would be more or less static. Estimates show, however, a continual increase from the earliest times for which data are available, down to the present day. Wars, plagues, famines and natural disasters represent only local and temporary setbacks. Moreover the increase is at an ever-accelerating rate.

Man is the only species that is multiplying in this way, and the reason is of course his ability to master the environment. Other species adapt to the environment, and slowly change their characteristics in the process; as was noted earlier, this is how new species originate. Man, however, has so conquered the environment that he has been able to spread all over the globe, and to thrive in every kind of climate. He has been able to do this without fundamental bodily changes; he has remained one species. In this he is unique.

He has also been able to nullify one after another the checks on his growth in numbers. He has improved his food-gathering and food-producing methods, he has protected himself against the elements, and he has controlled or eliminated many diseases. These processes scarcely seem yet to have reached the stage of diminishing returns; they have indeed accelerated prodigiously since the industrial revolution.

The obverse of the coin is that the environment is affected more and more drastically, as man's activities increase in scale and speed. This impact has moreover acquired new and significant characteristics. In earlier times man made use for the most part of natural products. There were some exceptions, but these were rare; the introduction of bronze and iron stands out so sharply that we speak of a Bronze Age and an Iron Age. Nowadays, however, new substances which never before existed on the earth are two a penny, and by various means they are spread around an environment that has never before had to cope with them. A few years ago, for example, detergents resistant to bacterial action produced great masses of drifting foam on some of our rivers, and they have had to be replaced by new 'bio-degradable' substances.

Another great change is in the amounts of energy at man's disposal. With modern machinery and explosives land can be levelled, forests cleared, bogs drained and rivers diverted on a scale unimaginable when man's principal power source was his own body and those of his domestic animals.

We have indeed reached a sombre stage of development. Man's power over the environment has grown to the point where he can actually destroy it; he can render the whole earth incapable of supporting life, and there is little in the contemporary scene to reassure us that his greed or folly will not cause this to happen. Many of his attitudes are inherited from earlier times, when he was less numerous and less powerful. Frequently his actions have been on a par with those of plants and animals, which simply exploit the environment for their own immediate benefit. Primitive man could afford to do this, but man armed with modern technology courts disaster unless he changes his ways.

Primitive man treated nature as if it were infinite in size, and modern man usually does the same. He behaves as if the atmosphere and the oceans were unlimited – inexhaustible supplies of air, water and salt, and capable of absorbing man's wastes in unrestricted quantities.

He also treats the mineral wealth of the world as if it were virtually inexhaustible. If a mine runs out, or an oil well runs dry he expects to find replacements. Similarly with the life of the seas: he hunts fish by increasingly sophisticated techniques, but without much thought for the consequences of overfishing. Yet overfishing is already with us, and as regards some kinds of whales extinction is a real danger.

The land, he has learned, is not inexhaustible. Nomads and primitive farmers were able in the past to keep moving on to fresh pastures and virgin lands, but population pressure is now almost everywhere too great for such modes of existence to be practicable. Settled farming usually requires some provision for renewal of the soil, and where this is neglected disasters like the North American 'dust-bowl' of the nineteen-thirties can be the result.

A more recent lesson, still only partially assimilated, is that wildlife cannot be regarded as limitless. Even in Africa it is necessary to establish nature reserves, and it may not be very long before some species of animals survive only in zoos.

Industrial countries like ours bear eloquent witness to the attitudes of our immediate forbears. Mines, factories and urban areas were established with little thought for amenity, beyond civic buildings and essential services. Natural landscapes were ruined and many rivers eventually degenerated into open sewers, all the fresh water being removed in the upper reaches and replaced by urban effluents.

Even when man's intervention is benign in its intention, and not merely heedless of the consequences, the results can be unfortunate. A classic case is that of the Kaibab deer of Arizona. A campaign was mounted to kill off the wolves, pumas and coyotes that preyed on the deer. The principal natural check on the deer population was thereby removed, and their numbers increased enormously, outrunning their food supply. Desperately trying to assuage their hunger, they browsed to higher and higher levels, to the detriment of the trees. Ultimately they died of starvation, and in much larger numbers than had ever been killed by predators.

Fortunately man's baneful influence is often mitigated by the self-regulating forces that create the balance of nature. The land, for example, usually recovers from over-grazing or over-cropping if left to itself for a few years, though there are limits to this process, as the deserts of North Africa bear witness.

Again, the atmosphere is self-cleansing. The smoke and the gaseous products we discharge are removed comparatively rapidly, mainly by rain and gravity, and are deposited on the surface of the land and the oceans, where they may even sometimes be beneficial. Rivers, too, are self-cleansing. The mud on their beds has a great capacity for absorbing noxious substances, both inorganic and organic. The oceans are even able to dispose of the oil discharged by ships, often illegally, on their surface, though the mechanisms concerned – dissolution and microbial action – require a certain time to take effect.

Nevertheless, despite the existence of these purifying and restoring processes, it is becoming less and less possible to leave the environment to look after itself in face of man's assaults. Protection, conservation and prevention of abuses are becoming increasingly necessary.

Pollution

There have been some dramatic demonstrations of the consequences of neglect in these matters. The London smog of 1952 will be remembered by many. Atmospheric conditions developed in which pollutants from homes, factories and traffic were trapped instead of dispersing, so that contamination rose to very high levels. The smog began on a Thursday and was cleared by wind and rain on the following Monday. The death rate in London on the Friday was well above normal, rose to a peak on the Monday, and remained high for at least a fortnight. In all, some 4,000 deaths are generally attributed to the smog. There is some, but not much, consolation in the thought that most of these 4,000 individuals were in poor health and might not have survived many months longer in any case.

The 1952 smog led to a Government enquiry, and that in turn led to the Clean Air Act of 1956 and increased research on air pollution. Implementation of the Clean Air Act has had dramatic results on visibility and air purity in London, Manchester, Sheffield and other cities. Although there was another major London smog in 1962, there is now good reason to hope that there will never be another of disaster proportions.

Los Angeles provides a smog story of a different kind. Here it is not a question of a few bad days in winter but of a chronic state of affairs, which is at its worst in summer. Trouble began rather abruptly in the early 1940's. The smog builds up according to a regular daily pattern, and it has the unpleasant property of causing lachrymation.

Los Angeles has spent more on air pollution problems than any other city in the world in its attempt to remove this blot on the Californian escutcheon. Ultimately it was discovered that the main culprit is automobile exhaust gases, acted on by the bright Californian sun; photochemical reactions take place, yielding the lachrymatory substances. The contamination hangs around in the still air between the sea and the mountains.

Smogs of the Los Angeles type are unlikely in Britain, because we are blessed with too little sun, but cities further south can expect them as motor vehicles increase in numbers. They have led to regulations with which all cars in North America must comply, and similar regulations may be expected in Europe.

There are no water pollution episodes quite as dramatic as the London and Los Angeles smog stories, yet most of the rivers in Britain's big cities have over the years become so contaminated as to be unable to sustain fish life. We have lived with this impoverishment of the environment for so long that we have come to take it for granted as part of the price of urbanisation. Yet it is not inevitable, and thanks to the unremitting efforts of the River Boards and others some of our rivers, including the Thames, are gradually being reclaimed.

Another major source of anxiety is the increasing use of chemicals on the farm. It is not always appreciated just how recently and how rapidly modern pesticides and herbicides have been introduced. Although inorganic poisons and natural products have been used much longer, the first synthetic products date back only to the last war, when DNOC was brought to Britain from France, the hormone weed-killers were developed in Britain, and DDT was smuggled in through occupied Europe from Switzerland. They were a godsend to a nation at war. Since then a couple of hundred more such products have been developed, many familiar to every gardener, and in the present decade their use has become the rule rather than the exception on British farms.

Of their positive achievements there can be no doubt, and in a world full of disease and malnutrition there are strong reasons for exploiting them to the full. An added inducement in a country like Britain is the way they save labour; indeed farmers would have been hard put to it to maintain production without them. Yet there is another side to the story. There has been a succession of episodes of dead animals, dead birds and dead fish; of valuable insects like bees being killed; of insect populations getting out of hand after their predators had been killed; of development of immunity to the new substances. While some of the new substances are destroyed by the soil and in other ways, others persist and can be passed from plant to insect to bird to carnivore, killing at each stage. Some tend, too, to accumulate in an animal, and they reach us in milk or meat. Pesticide residues are indeed now to be found almost everywhere, not excluding the air we breathe. Autopsies commonly reveal several parts per million of substances such as DDT in human corpses.

The situation is carefully watched in Britain by a variety of organisations, some official and some not. In particular there is a voluntary screening scheme for new agricultural products, to which all manufacturers submit. There are continual efforts to produce more acceptable products – less toxic to animals and birds, and less persistent. Nevertheless there is still cause for anxiety. The precautionary measures are concerned chiefly with the more immediate dangers; the long-term effects, for instance on the soil and on the general ecological balance, are receiving less attention.

The one threat to the environment that it can fairly be claimed has been exhaustively studied is that due to radioactivity. The world's introduction to the atomic age, through the atom bomb, produced a world-wide emotional reaction. There is as a result a really somewhat exaggerated fear of radioactivity, as compared with other hazards to man, but at least this has led to the most thorough research into all the health aspects, to the imposition of the most rigorous international controls, and to the most careful documentation of even the slightest degree of environmental contamination. Indeed we have in the handling of the problems of radioactivity a pattern that may usefully be applied to other pollutants.

Viewing the assaults on the environment as a whole, we have certainly little cause for complacency. Mushrooming world populations and accelerating technological progress combine to produce threats of damage to the environment that may prove irretrievable.

Conservation versus Exploitation

In Britain a great deal has been done in a fairly quiet way to meet the problems. Having led the world into the industrial revolution, we have also led the world in correcting some of its bad features. Other countries sometimes envy the success of our oddly-named Alkali Inspector in dealing with industrial effluents. Industry itself generally takes a responsible attitude. We have Government laboratories studying air and water pollution. We have various Ministries looking after amenities and setting standards. We have Nature Reserves, areas of outstanding natural beauty, and green belts. We have numerous private organisations which care about these things.

Yet it is still possible to ask if this is sufficient, and even if we think it is sufficient for our own country, whether we can be content to leave it at that.

Concern for the environment inevitably clashes with some of the demands of modern technology. It raises therefore fundamental issues about the kind of world we want to see. If we regard economics and modern technology as the most important things in the world, then we do not want the environment to stand in the way of what we call progress. Forests must be cleared, dams built and valleys flooded, power stations and pylons strung across the land, motorways and airports constructed. The danger is that each project is considered separately, and nobody attempts to assess the total effect on the environment. Objections to the project are usually of a local character, while the case in favour is presented in terms of its significance within some nationwide plan. A dam, for instance, may be put forward as an essential part of a national scheme for water and electricity supply. A false antithesis thereby appears between broad technological considerations and narrow environmental ones.

Moreover the economic advantage is usually all with the proposers of new plans, rather than with the objectors. Theirs is the profit-making side, and they have the resources to assemble and present their case in the most effective manner. At an enquiry they appear as impersonal champions of big projects benefiting many people, while their opponents are often in the position of defending personal interests. The latter are easily made to appear parochial and selfish, and we forget that the planner or the technical man, having put a great effort into devising his schemes, can be just as selfish in his own way, blind to alternatives, limited in outlook, and determined to force his plan through.

When battle is joined at a public enquiry, the issue is, for the reasons just given, pretty well decided in advance, though the objectors may win minor concessions. Occasionally, as in the case of the proposed Stanstead Airport, sufficient national attention is focused on the battle for it to take a different course, but this is exceptional.

It is doubtful whether the present-day weighting of the scales will be much changed without a change in our underlying philosophy. It is true that as we lose our amenities we learn to prize those that remain, and up to a point we are prepared to fight for them and pay for them. It is also true that we are developing concepts like 'social benefits' to throw into the scales, that is to say benefits that are so widely diffused that they do not appear directly in anyone's balance sheet. Nevertheless the effects of these factors look like being too little and too late. They are not radical enough in face of the materialism of our times. On every side nowadays we hear the cry that man has grown up, that he must accept his destiny and act like a god, bending the world to his will. It is small wonder that those who try to halt man's assaults on the environment often appear to be reactionaries. Often, too, they are associated with a sentimental and lopsided religious attitude.

This is unfair. The assertion that this is God's world, and that we should therefore respect and cherish the order of nature, and hesitate before we destroy anything in it, or even upset the ecological balance, is only one side of the picture. Christianity also asserts that man is ordained to be lord of nature. Animals, plants and minerals are there for man to use, and it is his duty to use them, responsibly, if he is to be his brother's keeper. Unfortunately, however, the two halves of this philosophy have usually got separated in modern life, and even appear in opposing camps.

Within the philosophy as a whole, there is ample room for both conservation and exploitation of the environment in the interests of science and technology. This does not mean that the two will always be easy to reconcile. Still less does it imply the existence of any simple universal formula which we can apply to each problem as it arises. What it does do is to assure us that the search for a reconciliation is always worth while and likely to be successful. It dissuades us from onesidedness in our approach. Moreover, since it is the Christian philosophy we are speaking of, it suggests that the key may be to find a higher wisdom than man's unaided reason can supply.

Primitive man grappled with difficult problems, and in so doing developed his brain and made possible the emergence of civilisation. It could be that modern man will reach a new stage of maturity as with God's help he finds responsible non-partisan answers to the problems created by his own proliferation and his own technology.

Further reading

BARRY COMMONER: 'Science and Survival' (Gollancz, 1966).
RACHEL CARSON: 'Silent Spring' (Hamish Hamilton, 1963).
JOHN COLEMAN-COOKE: 'The Harvest that Kills' (Odhams, 1965).

The author wishes to express his thanks to Dr. C. J. Banks, Dr. B. Loughman, Mr. K. Neal and Mr. G. N. Walton for their helpful comments.

Part Two

The Promotion of Health

5

THERAPY AND FAITH

Compiled by the Editors

Increasing importance is being attached to a 'multi-dimensional' approach to health. The need to bring together contributions from different branches of the medical profession has long been recognised, and there is a tendency nowadays to cast the net ever wider, drawing in such varied topics as welfare, marriage guidance and town and country planning. The creation of the science of ergonomics, in which engineering is harnessed to serve the needs of the human body, is a sign of the times.

Among all these developments the spiritual dimension must not be neglected. The Churches' Council on Healing exists indeed to make sure that full use is made of the therapeutic power of faith, and the Council of the British Medical Association has officially stated that 'there exists a field for legitimate and valuable co-operation between clergy and doctors in general and between the Churches' Council on Healing and the Association in particular'. They say furthermore that 'Medicine and the Church working together should encourage a dynamic philosophy of health which would enable every citizen to find a way of life based on moral principle and on a sound knowledge of the factors which promote health and well-being'.[1]

In broad general terms most people – even agnostics – would no doubt concede that religious beliefs often contribute to health, to patient acceptance of ill-health, and to

57

peace of mind in face of death. It is also true that doctors sometimes have occasion to appeal to a patient's faith in the course of treatment. What is rarer is for the doctor, or nurse, or anyone else concerned, to attempt to awaken faith in a patient who lacks it or has allowed it to fade.

When however this is attempted, the results are often remarkable and encouraging. Quite apart from miracles like those at Lourdes, there are many examples of the beneficial effects in the medical sphere of a patient's making contact with God. In this chapter a small selection of cases, drawn from various sources, has been assembled to illustrate the art. The hope may be expressed that those who read them may be inspired to fuller application of their own faith in their dealings with the sick.

A Rotten Doctor?

'I think you are a rotten doctor! I've been coming to you for over three months and you haven't done me any good at all.' This is what Arthur X said to me one day in the surgery when I had prescribed a change in medicine. 'In fact' he continued, 'the medical profession with all its advances is useless as far as I'm concerned. I've been going to you doctors on and off for years, I've had two operations, had all my teeth out and it's cost me a fortune. You're none of you any good.'

'Well, I don't think much of you as a patient,' I replied somewhat taken aback. 'You're no advertisement for me!' Then I thought that this pompous and rather stupid little man needed something drastic to shake him up realistically, to make him face himself and his stupidity. I blazed at him, 'If you would carry out my instructions you would soon be better. I put you on a diet – you don't stick to it. I told you to cut out smoking – you are still doing it. I forbade alcohol which irritates your stomach – but you continue. I very much doubt if you take your medicine regularly.'

I expected an explosion, but I had hit home. The poor little man looked deflated. He had never been spoken to like that before. I followed up my advantage by saying, 'You are quite right, the medical profession can do nothing for you!'

There was an awkward silence between us and then, 'You are quite right. Thank God I've found an honest doctor at last!'

He was an architect, aged 49. He was employed to supervise the building of post offices and telephone exchanges and had moved about from place to place, so that as his health was poor he had been under a number of different doctors in various towns. He suffered from a duodenal ulcer, but on account of his nervous disposition was troubled by sleeplessness, palpitations and headaches. He had been fully investigated in hospital by X-rays, test meals and so on. Small of stature, like many such, he compensated by aggressiveness. He was short tempered and impatient. Untidy in appearance, he always looked worried. He had a characteristic frown which had become chronic. You could tell at a glance that nothing seemed to go right for him. There was always something wrong; if it wasn't the weather, it was the neighbours; if not the neighbours, it was the government or the men on the building site!

He had consulted me about three months before and I had been treating him on traditional lines, recognising that his complaint was largely nervous, though it had an organic manifestation.

'Tell me, doctor,' he asked, 'what will cure me if you can't?'

'You need to manage yourself, break your habits and discipline yourself as well as your diet and indulgences,' I replied.

'It's all very well,' he responded, 'but a drink and a smoke take off the irritations of life and make it bearable. I get so worried and have so many difficulties that I must have some relief.'

I knew that his home was not happy and his staff detested him. It was no use arguing with him; I would have won the argument and left him all the more resentful and frustrated.

'Tell me,' I said, 'what would you do if your car kept going wrong and the local garages couldn't put it right?'

'Send it back to the maker,' came the reply.

After a pause, I hinted, 'Well, that's what you have got to do – go back to your Maker.'

C

'Oh,' said he, 'but I'm an atheist,' as if that let him out. 'Have you ever made a mistake in your life?' I asked.

'Fair enough,' he laughed, 'What do I do?' I said, 'Why not pray a prayer like this? – O God, if you are, please manage me and tell me what to do because I can't manage myself.' This was a novel idea. 'All right,' he agreed, 'I'll try anything once.' So we sat in the surgery and he prayed that prayer, saying it slowly after me. Then we were quiet, I suppose for about two minutes. 'Well, what happened?' I asked. 'Nothing,' he answered, 'I didn't hear a voice or anything.' 'God speaks,' I said, 'through our thoughts.' 'Oh,' he remarked, 'I had plenty of thoughts, but nothing relevant.' 'Tell me about them,' I enquired. 'Well,' he said, 'If you want to know, I was thinking about a subordinate of mine at the office. He is a bumptious, self-opinionated young man and I always enjoyed taking him down a peg. I sent him out this morning to survey a site; he made a hopeless mess of it and returned without the details we required. I rebuked him for incompetence and laziness. It occurred to me, however, that if I had given him the necessary information, he could have done the job. That's all – you see there was nothing relevant, nothing about my ulcer.'

'Now,' I reminded him, 'you prayed to God to show you what to do. Suppose there happens to be a God, and He happens to be Love and Truth, do you think that He might have been suggesting to you that your action in withholding the information and then rebuking your subordinate was neither loving nor truthful.'

'Good heavens,' he gasped, 'if that's God speaking, I've heard Him before.' Then, after a moment, 'If I'm to be loving and truthful, I'll have to apologise, give the man the facts and let him have another try.'

He came again the next evening. It had been difficult to eat humble pie, but he had apologised and given the essential facts and figures to his young colleague, who had returned this time with the job perfectly done. 'And,' he added, 'he's not such a bad chap after all!'

He had restored a relationship and learned a secret. He started to test his behaviour by love and truth and make them a target for all he did. There was a lot of clearing up to do. He tackled his home first. He asked his wife to forgive him for his coldness and lack of caring. There were no children. He had refused her opportunity. He was full of resentment against her because, amongst other things, both her old parents had spent their last days in his home. Their illnesses had been expensive and he had had to pay for the funerals. He was living beyond his income, was full of fear that his health would break down, forcing early retirement on an inadequate pension. His life was in a mess; resentment, fear and dishonesty played havoc with his glands and system. No wonder he was ill. Now, however, he found a new way of life, a purpose, a golden thread to which he could cling. His wife forgave him and together they started to reshape their lives. They tackled their spending. Because he saw it was dishonest to spend so much on his drinks and smokes when he was overdrawn at the bank and stingy with the housekeeping allowance, he decided to cut them out. He began to be strict with his diet and regular with his medicine. He found his worries at the office resolved with the new relationships that came through his different behaviour. In a matter of weeks he lost his symptoms. He began to be more cheerful, and he looked different because he was coming to terms with life.

One day when he came to see me for a routine consultation, I could see there was something bothering him. His frown had come back. There was trouble on the building site. There was a walk out. He said they were behindhand with the work and he feared the penalties if the job was not completed by the contract date. The men, he said, had downed tools. 'Why?' I asked. 'I don't know,' he said. 'They're a lazy lot – I wish you would come and talk to them.' 'Don't be ridiculous,' I said, 'That's your job.' I found he had never taken any interest in them; he did not know their names or anything about them. He soon saw what he could do to find out what the trouble was, so on the way back he dropped in on the foreman instead of waiting for the formal visit which had been arranged. He found it was a storm in a teacup. Since demolishing an outhouse in preparation for further buildings, the men had had nowhere to leave their bicycles which became drenched when left out in the rain. His reputation was such that no one dared to approach him even though it was such a trifling detail. He immediately blamed them for their stupidity, but a moment's thought showed him how his lack of interest and caring had produced the impasse. He had learned the secret of apology and in no time the situation was resolved. He told his foreman to make a temporary shed with timber and corrugated iron. That afternoon he personally walked round and talked to the men explaining about the work and taking an interest in them. One of them was a friend of a patient of mine who told me all about it. 'The bloke's different,' he said.

Day by day each morning Arthur and his wife would listen to the voice within, which gave them direction and balance for the day. The things they used to quarrel about like the garden, her housekeeping allowance, entertaining his colleagues and her friends, became opportunities to discover the right plan. Life became real and purposeful. His overdraft began to sink, he set himself a target to liquidate it, his health improved, he slept better, no longer did he worry about the future, he had new friends whom he helped to find a way of life that satisfied.

In three months his ulcer healed. People remarked on his changed appearance. The work progressed and was finished on time. The day the job was finished, he came to see me to thank me for his recovery. I said, 'There is no need to thank me, you want to thank God.' 'I do,' he said simply. 'So you believe in Him?' 'Believe in Him?' he said. 'I know Him.'

E.C.

Problems of Relationships

When I first met Mr Jones, he was fifty years old. Naturally stern, his face had a haggard look. Slightly stooped, he seemed older than his years; and his eyes, when he took off his glasses were tired and worried. His feet shifted restlessly as he talked.

For seven years, he told me, he had had arthritic pains. These had slowly increased but had, apparently, been of no permanent damage to any of his joints. His sedimentation index was 0.9. He had lost some thirty pounds!

His relationship history disclosed a deep-seated resentment against some of his business associates, and his home relationships were strained. Although quite successful in business, he had a sense of complete failure about his whole life. He was desperately anxious to find an answer to these frustrations, but his inherited religion was undeveloped and superficial and in no way met his needs or affected his actions.

The usual medical regimen was started. His first spiritual step was to face the truth about himself, going over each failure honestly, in detail, and asking forgiveness for it, in order completely to leave the past behind and make a fresh start. Then we began his spiritual education; he studied the Bible and took time to think through its teachings. As soon as he understood and accepted one of the spiritual laws, he put it into action. He apologized to his associates for his jealousy and resentments and put things right at home.

During the first year there was a complete change in Mr Jones's physical health. He gained back his weight and his arthritic condition cleared up except for occasional stiffness of his neck and lame arches. His sedimentation index came down to 0.5. During the next twenty years he was free from all joint symptoms.

His spiritual foundations had been firmly laid and were the basis for his conduct. Because of his changed attitude the whole family relationship was extremely happy, with a return of co-operation and affection. He brought a new spirit to his job and was able to help many of his associates, finding that the best way to keep his experience fresh and vital was to pass it on.

From LORING T. SWAIM: 'Arthritis, Medicine and the Spiritual Laws' (Blandford, 1963), pp. 59–60.

... Then there was Betsy, who at least twice a year paid me a series of visits, usually before Christmas and early in June. Sometimes the complaint was that she was just too tired to work and that she was afraid she was going to have colitis. Sometimes she said she had colitis again and was too tired to work. Each time at some point she would raise the question about her job, perhaps she was in the wrong one. She wasn't especially happy. What did I think she ought to do about it?

At other times she came in just to be examined to be sure she didn't have cancer, or tuberculosis. If one of her friends developed any serious illness, Betsy was sure to drop in to see me in a few days to find out whether she was not the victim of the same disorder.

Rest and diet would always relieve her colitis, but never give her peace of mind. She was just about immune to the idea that faith might cure her fears, though all her life she had lived in the bosom of the church.

As a child she went to church twice on Sundays and several times during the week. Her father was a prosperous coal merchant in a small upstate city (in the U.S.A.), and his life and that of her mother was centred in the local Episcopal church where he was church warden and super-intendent of the Sunday School, and she was a leading worker in all the women's organisations.

Betsy, an only child, had a happy, protected childhood and was devoted to her parents. On her graduation from college they suggested she fit herself for religious education. She acquiesced readily enough. Anyway, she expected to get married and one job was as good as another until that happened. Only she didn't get married and at forty she was a notable authority on religious education and head of a large staff of teachers in a city church. Thanks to her father's generosity she was always well dressed. She appeared poised and graciously helpful, but at times her inner fears over-whelmed her and she felt the need of medical help.

One day I took her health record for the previous seven years out of the file and went over it with her.

'You've had colitis fifteen times in the past seven years, more often in June and December. It's curious, isn't it?'

'Yes,' she said, 'although I also had it badly when I was home last March for my aunt's operation. I was very worried about her.'

I continued. 'You've always associated these symptoms

with worry. Now I would like you to think about what is so intolerable in your life that you can't face it. What is worse just before Christmas and before vacation? I suspect you know in your heart.'

After a while she began to cry.

'I can't stand these complacent women with their spoiled children. I have to visit them on Christmas and be on hand for all church festivities. I always get out of it if I can.'

Another pause, and then, 'I suppose I would like to be in their shoes myself. I hate being an old maid and I dread that month at home. When Aunt Ella was so sick last year I was afraid if she died I would have to go home to live.'

When she finally calmed down I said I would like to ask her one more question. 'Whom do you love?'

With great reluctance at last she said: 'I suppose only myself. I can't think of anyone else. How very awful! If I can't have a husband I won't care about anyone at all. No wonder my stomach stops functioning!'

She was a long time getting over her symptoms, but we were on the right track. The trouble was really in her heart and not her digestive tract. When Aunt Ella got ill again and her mother had a heart attack at the same time, she went home. To her amazement she loved running the house, caring for the older people. She wrote me that she never had time to be ill.

From IRENE GATES: 'Any Hope, Doctor?' (Blandford, 1954), pp. 120–22.

One of my patients was an engineer called Bert. He worked at a bench in a large factory. He was always attending the surgery for common ailments and minor conditions, colds, bronchitis, influenza, 'lumbago' and such like. He bitterly complained of the factory conditions where he said that no one was happy, he was cold and he worked in a draught. This, he said, was the reason for his poor health. 'Why not get the management to put the conditions right?' I asked. He said it was impossible, he had constantly complained to the foreman who was such a b . . . but his complaint was never heard, and he doubted whether it had even reached the shop superintendent.

It was clear that there was no love lost between these two men. Bert was full of hatred, bitterness and jealousy. I pointed out to him that this was what was spoiling his life and lay behind his various illnesses. He said, 'Yes, I know, but what can I do?' 'Why not make friends with him?' I asked. There was no reply. 'What do you think you ought to do?' I enquired. 'Have you anything to apologise to him for?' 'I can't do that,' he replied. 'He'd think me soft.' 'You are soft,' I said. 'You haven't the guts to admit where you have been wrong.'

This stung Bert to action. A few days later he was back in the surgery – this time all smiles. He told me he had done it; the foreman was so surprised that he, in his turn, apologised to him for having done nothing about the heating and draught. Together they had approached the management. The superintendent was so surprised to see these proverbial rivals working together that he listened to their advice about the heating and ventilation of the floor and saw that the necessary changes were made.

I did not see him for some weeks, and when I met him in the road he told me that peace reigned in the factory, that he and the foreman had become good friends, and that the atmosphere at work had improved and production had gone up. He had discovered that to do what his heart and conscience bade him made life different all round. He decided to give up smoking because he said he knew that was why he had a cough and bronchitis. The money saved could now be spent on home and family. This discovery had not only improved his health but had given him a faith or philosophy of life and a happiness at home which they surely needed. More than that, it had improved the health and happiness of the workers on the shop floor.

E.C.

Drug Addiction

M. was a drug addict admitted to my surgical ward for treatment of abscesses which had occurred as a result of injecting herself with dirty needles. She was completely 'hooked', and a very repulsive specimen of humanity. The doctor in charge told students, 'That girl will be dead in two years,' and regarded her as beyond hope or help.

Yet when she told her story of how she had started on drugs – the boredom, uncertainty and unhappiness that are not uncommon among young people today – there was something very lost and pathetic about her that went straight to the heart. Three of us in the hospital, all committed Christians, decided with God's help to give her a purpose to live for. We had to be practical about it as she was one of many other patients, and we had to start from where she was. Drug addicts have no sense of right and wrong, and will lie, cheat and steal to obtain their drugs.

We told her that God had power to free her from drugs and to give her a purpose in life far more fascinating than anything she could imagine. These would have been just empty words if God had not been real to us; if we had not found from Him the power to be loving and firm, patient and compassionate; if there had been no difference in our own lives to which M. could respond. M. had to see something in us, before she could begin to want something new for herself.

There was no instantaneous miracle, and many ups and downs, but as we became friends M. began to regain her self-respect. She was with us for six weeks and in that time she came off all drugs. We got in touch with other people after she left us, who could continue the caring we had started. Nine months after she was admitted, a physical, mental and moral wreck, to my ward, she returned to live at home and took a job as a hairdresser.

Contributed by a Nursing Sister

In my new form at school in Scandinavia in 1967 there were two hippies. They believed they could be happier by living simply, with a minimum of material goods; their slogan was 'Make love, not war'; and narcotics had a great part in their lives. I was fascinated and decided to try their way of life, although I knew that the consequences could be serious if the police found out. I did not give a thought to the effect on my mentality or my body. Even when later my friends and family said I had become apathetic and strange, I did not believe them.

The two hippies meanwhile had hitchhiked to India, thinking to find a poorer, simpler society where it would be easier for them to live in accordance with their ideas. They sent us letters occasionally from different places. Then suddenly there was a telegram from one of them saying he was seriously ill and asking us to send money to pay a doctor. We started a fund, but it had not got very far before a further telegram arrived from the German Embassy in Nepal. Our young friend had died from an infection from a dirty L.S.D. needle.

At the same time the police moved in on our drug-ring. Many of my friends were rounded up early in the morning and questioned for hours at the police-station. I was afraid one of them would mention my name, so I went away from home.

Later that week the other young man came home from the East, seriously ill with jaundice. He spent a long time in hospital, but they could not do much for him, and he has only five to ten years to live at best.

Finally in the same week I was expelled from school. My teachers were fed up, because the drugs had made me unresponsive, attending only when I felt like it and doing my homework only if I thought it interesting.

At the end of it all I felt terribly depressed. My whole world had fallen to pieces. I just sat down and cried like a little child until slowly I realised that I had to make a new beginning and that I had to finish with drugs or they would finish me. But it is one thing to see what you ought to do and another to break your dependence on drugs.

Some of my friends sought medical help, but doctors can only assist up to a certain point, and then it is up to the patient whether he is going to be cured or not. So long as his motive in life is to find an easy way out of his difficulties, he is likely to go back on to drugs again.

In my case some friends who knew my situation invited me to Switzerland with them to cheer me up again. I was glad just to get away from the mess I had made of things. A few days later I was lifted right out of my little corner. By chance I made my way to the Moral Re-Armament centre at Caux, where I met people from many nations with a bigger vision of what was happening in the world than I had ever had, and a determination to do something constructive about it. I grasped at what they had to offer because I realised it could save me – it could give me something worthwhile to do with my life. I felt I was needed and that I could perhaps help other people.

I thought it would be very difficult to stop using drugs, and even cigarettes, but in fact, having now a real purpose in life, I found it easy to make a clean break. I made the decision during a half-hour wait at a railway station. I walked up and down the platform really enjoying my last cigarette, and when I had finished I said to myself, 'All right, that's it. From now on you are never going to take tobacco or drugs again.'

I used not to have much of a faith, but I am beginning to find one. I think God really helped me when I needed Him most. One of my best friends died young because of drugs and another is going to die, but by a miracle I stopped in time. Many young people can be saved if they get the right sort of challenge. For me rehabilitation succeeded because it came from God.

For obvious reasons the writer of this account wishes to remain anonymous

Facing Death

The man in the bed opposite mine was clearly very ill. He was old, his face was ashen, he was unable to eat food, he coughed up blood. The parson on his visit to the ward, stood at the foot of the bed and told this man how much better he was looking. 'You'll soon be A1 at Lloyd's, he concluded. The sick man seemed to be neither convinced nor comforted.

It seemed to me that a fellow patient, whatever his limitations, had a better opportunity to share the faith he had found, than a visitor who tried to say a word of good cheer to all in the ward. So I slipped over to the old man's bed-side.

'When I had my heart attack,' I said, 'I was so ill that I couldn't do anything for myself. I had to trust the doctors and nurses to do everything for me.'

'I'm like that now,' was the reply.

'You know,' I went on, 'the doctors didn't ask if I was a good man or a bad man. They just did their best for me, as I was, because that is what they were there to do and what they wanted to do.'

My friend nodded assent.

'Have you ever thought of our Heavenly Father being like that?' I continued.

There was a silence for a while. Then the old man said: 'My wife used to talk like that, a long while ago.'

Then, after more silence, he went on: 'If God is like that, it doesn't matter much, does it, which world we are in?'

It was my turn to nod assent. And I added: 'To enable the doctors to do their best for me, I had to co-operate with them and go on the régime they suggested. For God to be able to do His best for me, I have willingly put himself under His régime. And that, for me, meant a lot of change.'

My friend did not get well but he was at peace as he put his hand in the Hand of God.

Contributed by Roger Hicks

Norman G. was an old gentleman of seventy who was dying of cancer of the bladder. He was a most difficult case to nurse. His bed was always wet. The district nurse who came twice a day and his wife were quite worn out. He was afraid of cancer and of dying and his wife and family would not let him be told the truth about his illness.

Eventually he asked me if he had got cancer. I told him that I thought that there were worse things than cancer. 'Oh,' he said, 'what could be worse than that?' I replied that I thought that not knowing God and His plan for me must be worse. He was thoughtful for a moment and then he said, 'If I knew God's plan for my life – it wouldn't matter so much if I did have cancer.' Then he added, 'How can I find God's plan?' I said, 'Ask Him – begin by putting right anything that you know in your heart is wrong.'

He told me that there were two things on his conscience. One was a business deal where he had taken advantage of an unwitting client and the other was that he felt so cross with his wife who got angry with him over his wet bed and his many complainings. I said that God would show him what to do about these two problems. He thought and then said, 'I could square up with Mr Jones and send him a cheque, and I could ask Annie to forgive me for being so cross and demanding.' He did both these things.

When I called next day the sick room was transformed. His apology to his wife had begun to restore their broken relationship. They had sat up talking half the night clearing up the little things that had come between them because of the shadow of his illness. He told her that he knew that he could not recover (though no one had told him this). They talked over his business affairs and he had made his will. From that time he became peaceful and co-operative over his nursing. It was the beginning of a new life for them both. They found a faith. God became real to them. They even helped their neighbours by passing on their experience. People who came to visit and bring flowers left his home uplifted and challenged by the change in them both. The day he died, some six weeks later, he said to me, 'I thank God for this illness. Without it I would never have known this peace.'

E.C.

A Letter from Mr Wong

'Dear Dr Swaim: The story is enclosed. You may use it in any way you see fit. I shall be most grateful to God if my personal experience can be helpful to some doctors somewhere and some day in the future.

'I was born to a reasonably wealthy family in Shanghai. My father is an atheist, my mother a Buddhist and I was brought up under Confucius's teachings. Being educated in an Episcopal university, aside from regular engineering courses I had the opportunity of studying the Bible every Sunday. Although I was impressed by the Gospel and amazed by the many similarities between the teaching of Jesus and Confucius, I always felt that it was silly to believe in a supernatural power in this modern world of science.

'In 1940, I was fortunate in obtaining a scholarship for advanced studies at Harvard University. The scholarship covered my tuition and my family supplied my living expenses. After the first year of study, I earned my Master's degree and I was well on my way towards the Doctorate. Then came the horrible Pearl Harbor incident in December 1941 and my funds from home were cut off. At first I tried to make ends meet by taking odd jobs at the school but that was not sufficient. Instead I had to seek work in Boston and devote nights to my thesis. By June 1942, being constantly worried about my future as well as the safety of my parents and suffering the effects of malnutrition, I finally succumbed to an attack of spondylitis, the form of arthritis you called Strümpell-Marie, that affected my spine and hip, producing excruciating pains with each step I took.

'Under the auspices of Harvard, I was admitted to a general hospital in Boston where my legs were put under traction, but the pain persisted each time I tried to take a step. At first lots of friends came to visit me, but as time went by they began to turn to other things. Lying flat on my back day in and day out, worrying and wondering, I could not help but feel sorry for myself. Many a night I silently cried myself to sleep.

'After two months I was transferred to the Robert Brigham Hospital where I met you. At that time, I was almost flat broke, but you took my case anyway. My body was put in a plaster cast and physiotherapy prescribed. You stopped by my bedside and chatted with me whenever you were in the ward. It was indeed gratifying to find a doctor who cared for me as a human being rather than as a part of his daily routine. I was slowly improving but I still could not throw off my deep anxiety about my future, my schoolwork and so forth.

'One day after your rounds, you came to me to have our usual chat, at which I expressed my impatience about my slow recovery and you assured me that I was progressing satisfactorily. It was at the end of that conversation that you said something to me which changed my entire life and which I shall never forget. You said, "Charlie, you and I are only human, why don't you trust yourself to God a little more?"

'That night when everybody in the ward was asleep, I prayed to God. For the first time out of my own volition, I told the Lord about all my fears and troubles and promised that I would trust in Him. Then for some reason fragments of the 23rd Psalm came into my mind. I recited, "The Lord is my shepherd; I shall not want. He maketh me to lie down in green pastures; He leadeth me beside the still waters . . ." and then I fell asleep and had the soundest sleep in many a month.

'The next morning I woke up refreshed and took my first step without spasmodic pain. From that day on I prayed every night and my improvement was miraculous.

'Immediately after being released from the hospital, I found a job in New York with a boss who understood my physical handicap. After attending services in churches of various denominations, I finally decided to join the Marble Collegiate Church and was baptized there.

'It has been over seventeen years since I found God at the hospital. In the interim, I changed jobs, married the most wonderful girl in my life, fathered two intelligent children and was able to live a normal life. Once in a while, my back will hurt a little, the hip not at all, but I have learned to live with it as I believe that it is God's warning for me, whenever it comes, to slow down my activities a bit.'

Dr. Swaim adds the following comment:

In April 1960 Mr and Mrs Wong brought their two children to visit us. I had a chance to examine him. Usually after twenty years Strümpell-Marie arthritis fuses the whole spine and bows the back over, causing loss of motion in the chest and sometimes in the hips. Mr Wong wore a plaster jacket for several years to correct his posture, prevent this bowing, and stop strain on his hips. As a result, today he moves his neck and hips and can expand his chest $1\frac{1}{2}$ inches. His posture is good, allowing him to hold a responsible business position.

From LORING T. SWAIM: 'Arthritis, Medicine and the Spiritual Laws' (Blandford, 1963), pp. 83–5.

REFERENCE

(¹) 'Medicine and the Church'. *British Medical Journal*, 8 November 1947, p. 112

6

REHABILITATION

M. H. M. HARRISON, CH.M., B.M., CH.B., F.R.C.S.

Mr Max Harrison is Consultant Surgeon to the Royal Orthopaedic Hospital, Birmingham, the General Hospital, Birmingham, and the Robert Jones and Agnes Hunt Orthopaedic Hospital, Oswestry.

Rehabilitation means helping a patient to achieve the highest level of living of which he is capable. Such a level is not relative to that of other people and certainly bears no relation to any supposed 'normal'; it is the maximum that can be conceived as possible for this patient at this time. 'At this time' indicates the dynamic nature of the concept. Other levels may be reached in the future. Every patient requires rehabilitation and every doctor requires to make himself responsible for directing the rehabilitation programme.

Our ideas on the subject owe a great deal to Sir Reginald Watson-Jones' work with the Royal Air Force during the Second World War. His writings conveyed most graphically how service personnel could be restored to one hundred per cent fitness after serious injury, as their minds and bodies were given a progressive restoration through the talents of doctor, gymnast, physiotherapist and welfare officer. 'Treatment' included buoyant company, games, social pastimes, the sound of the lark and the sight of the heather. A will to overcome was fostered and the way to triumph was shown.

To make rehabilitation practical requires understanding between the doctor and his patient. At every meeting of doctor and patient the former makes an evaluation of the latter. Sometimes this is done after a lengthy process of questioning, listening, clinical examination using all the senses, laboratory and other special investigations. Sometimes, particularly at consultations other than the first, the evaluation can be made within a few minutes. The more skilled and experienced the doctor, the quicker and more accurate may be his assessment. This is what we mean by diagnosis. Having made a diagnosis the next desirable step is treatment which often consists in exposing the patient to one or more physical influences designed to combat or reverse the disease process. What else? The need for something more can readily be sensed by the relative of a sick person who asks the patient on his return from a visit to the doctor, 'Well, what did he say?' The answer is so often, 'Nothing really, just to carry on and see him again in three weeks, and he gave me another certificate.'

'Explaining to the patient' is often omitted in a busy practice these days; explanations certainly are required but they do not of necessity meet the need outlined in the conversation quoted above. The doctor's explanations should not be based on physiological or pathological concepts which even an intelligent layman often fails to grasp, let alone a nervous and ill person. Even when explanations are conveyed successfully, the patient who understands what the doctor believes to be causing his symptoms may still not have discovered what he wants to know. For example, a patient suffering from sciatica can be told, 'Your pain is due to something irritating a nerve in your back'. Not infrequently today the patient replies, 'Is it a slipped disc, doctor?' An honest answer to this question would probably be, 'I don't know', or "You will have to decide whether I am too stupid or too honest to answer that question!' But the clue to the type of approach we are considering is to be found in, 'What you really want to know, isn't it, is what is to be done to get you right?' As this phrase is comprehended the anxious look gives way to an emphatic and relieved, 'Yes, that is right, Doctor.'

Targets for the Patient's Recovery

Every time a doctor sits down with his patient he should set a target. When the patient leaves the doctor he should have quite clearly within his sights what he is to achieve and by when. A person who has just had a Colles' fracture of the wrist reduced and plastered is told to regain full finger motion and retain full shoulder range. This will take some doing, and help from a physiotherapist is important because, although failure of the broken bone to join is unheard of, painful stiff fingers and shoulders are ten a penny. When the patient is seen again the doctor checks whether the target has been reached, expresses his approval and congratulations if it has, and if not, finds out why. Fear, pain, laziness, ignorance, resentment are possible reasons for failure. The cause must be diagnosed and dealt with. When the target has been achieved a new one is set.

Target thinking is valuable in physiotherapy. A woman tripped on an uneven paving stone and in falling cut and contused her knee. The wound was expertly stitched and later because of knee pain and weakness she was given a great deal of physiotherapy including massage and electrical treatments of several types. Persisting pain and weakness amounted to a substantial disability and in pursuing legal damages she was referred for an opinion on her future. The opinion was expressed that her trouble was due to muscle weakness and that physiotherapy should be able to restore muscle power and remove her symptoms. The woman protested that she had already had hours of treatment without benefit. The remedy lay in setting a target. The power in the weak muscle was estimated by recording the maximum weight she could lift ten times, and was compared with the normal knee – 2 lb. against 20 lb. She was advised to attend the Physiotherapy Department thrice weekly and to do as much repetitive exercise at home as would raise the weight from 2 lb. to 4 lb. in one week. This she achieved, still felt no better, but now had hope of improvement. Weekly power checks showed a progressive increase and in six weeks the damaged knee was stronger than the other one and her disability had gone. Concentration on reaching targets rather than on abolishing symptoms ensured a complete rehabilitation. Her legal compensation was less but she was delighted.

Return to Work

To continue the previous example of the Colles' fracture, the injured person can be moved up to a higher level of living – rehabilitated – by getting to work. The doctor will have to enquire about the patient's normal work – be it housewife or factory fitter – and be knowledgeable enough to know how such work can be modified. He then tells the patient, 'I want you to get on with your housework. You can do absolutely anything with this wrist as long as you keep the plaster dry. You won't do the fracture any harm at all, indeed it will do it the world of good.' This advice is now known to be scientifically accurate. 'The more you use it the better it will be. I will see you in five weeks and remove the plaster and I want to see some evidence that you have been working hard.' A factory worker spoken to in similar terms may well be able to return to his pre-accident work; others may clearly need to have their work modified or alternative employment provided. This latter step, requiring confidence between doctor, patient and employer, is much more difficult than the mechanics of fracture reduction and fixation. The skills of the Medical Social Worker and Disabled Resettlement Officer are of great assistance here. They may be required again when the broken wrist is removed from plaster and pronounced joined, and a new target is set. The patient is again told what he can do and a further appointment made at which it can be checked that he has in fact done it, and a further target set. The process is continued until maximum living has been obtained.

I am indebted to Mr L. W. Plewes, Director of the Accident Service of the Luton and Dunstable Hospital, for many of the viewpoints expressed in this chapter, for at Luton one sees rehabilitation working very effectively. Five days after removal of a knee cartilage Plewes' patient takes his place in the Vauxhall Motor Company production line. Removal of stitches and later follow-up examinations are conducted by the surgeon in the factory and even on the production line. These patients are at ease in their normal daily surroundings, and as they are not attending hospital, they do not 'feel ill'. For those for whom suitable work cannot be found, places are made available in the Hospital's Rehabilitation Centre or for Vauxhall employees in the factory's own centre built by the Company under the direction of Plewes.

The centre consists of an industrial workshop under the control and management of a skilled engineer. Patients are given tasks carefully selected to fit both the disability and the needs of each patient; for example a person recovering from an attack of sciatica, whose back is stiff and requires mobilising, operates a hand press cutting wire into short lengths. This forces him to bend down and pick up a length of wire, insert it into the machine and then bring down the handle, the operation being repeated many hundred times each day. As his treatment progresses the lengths of wire are placed at levels progressively lower than bench height and the press is moved further away from him thus gradually stretching and mobilising his spine. Treatment or work? The workshop is producing articles for the commercial market, the patient feels useful, his doubts and fears have vanished, and he soon returns to his own place of work.

After injury or illness a return to work is a useful final target; in a Welfare State this needs some emphasis because certain factors tend to operate against this goal. From many different sides we are informed of the desirability of leisure and of multiple avenues whereby it can be explored. By implication work may seem relatively undesirable and after illness or injury it may seem only just that the patient should, at any rate for a time, enjoy the former at the expense of the usual work routine. However, in reality a period off work often operates to the patient's disadvantage and should it become a protracted experience, irreversible damage may be done to his personality. At worst, and this is by no means uncommon, he may never be able to return to work again owing to the gradual accumulation of certain symptoms. Whether these are in part subconscious expressions of various fears of the ultimate return may be debateable; what is borne out by experience is that work is good medicine.

In this connection there is clearly doubt in the minds of some who advise patients who are entitled to or seeking legal damages. Frequently the claimants receive direct or implied suggestions to stay away from work with a view to increasing the damages they may receive. In my opinion this is wrong. The inability-to-work attitude, maintained for long periods, may become so entrenched in the patient's personality as to aggravate his disability, often permanently. I was involved in a medico-legal dispute concerning the honesty of a claimant who two years after severe injury (fractured spine, elbow and foot) complained of back-ache incapacitating him to a considerable degree. The fact that this man had returned to his pre-accident work only seven weeks after receiving these injuries was an eloquent testimony to his drive and genuineness. A settlement was achieved in his favour.

Permanent Disablement

For the patients described so far the target is the restoration of pre-accident normality. It is not always so. In 1957 at the Rancho los Amigos Hospital, Downey, California there was a ward in which all the patients were in artifical respirators. They were unable to breathe as a result of the ravages of severe infantile paralysis. The man responsible for preserving them alive was Vernon Nickel, an orthopaedic surgeon in many ways years ahead of his time. A pioneer of what a visiting surgeon in admiration called 'scrap-heap surgery', he expressed private doubts – 'Is it worth it? Sometimes I feel tempted to kick off the switch'. The Christmas after my visit I received a Christmas card which alone I remember of all those I have ever received. An etching of three choristers against a background of a church window, it was delicately beautiful. A note on the inside described how it was drawn by one of the patients just described whose body was totally paralysed but who held the pencil in her teeth. This is living to the maximum, a successful rehabilitation programme for a maximally paralysed person. Worth while? A Christmas card which can make one healthy recipient question the calibre of his living – yes, definitely worthwhile. Good work, Rancho.

Michael G. is one of my favourite patients. 'Arthrogryposis multiplexa congenita' means many stiff joints present from birth. Michael is a marked example. Dislocated hips, bent knees, downward pointing feet, stiffish elbows and wrists, with double ruptures and too tight a stomach exit (congenital pyloric stenosis) thrown in for good measure.

His handsome young mother was understandably daunted by this travesty of her expectations and wished him to be kept in hospital; undoubtedly the sort of baby that the abortion lobby would see best destroyed before birth. An early operation freed his digestive tube and then the target was to get him ready to stand. I started on his lower limbs. Moderate success after operations planned to bring his feet plantigrade were followed by failure to straighten the knees by plaster or surgical techniques. Walking would clearly be impossible and eventually I contemplated the amputation of both legs through the knee joints and providing artificial limbs. A second opinion from another colleague suggested a last-ditch radical and rather different approach. The removal of each ankle bone and division of every structure round the knees except one artery, vein and nerve got the limbs straight.

Michael is now aged 5, walks with leg irons, attends an ordinary infant school, has a smile that would melt an ogre's heart, and is an immense source of joy to his mother and all medical and nursing personnel who encounter him. You feel better for knowing him. His future? What of yours? A triumphant personality whose every act is inspiring.

The Importance of Motivation

In rehabilitation so much depends on motives, as of course it does in all human relationships. Does the patient feel that his doctor really cares for him or merely sees him as a unit? This will condition his response to the suggestion that he returns to modified duties. Does the employer care enough for the workman to face the inconvenience and risk of accommodating the patient before he is one hundred per cent fit? Those employers who have done so have earned bonuses in improved labour-management relationships which can never be conferred by bargaining. Does the doctor understand the value and dignity of work in his own life, so that he understands how he must strive to encourage his patient to return and the employer to accept him? How much easier it is to give off-work certification and to keep repeating it. In the long run the doctor's personal standards may help to decide community attitudes to these problems.

Rehabilitation is a matter of goals and of motivation, a moral question and not one of departments and physical resources. We train medical students in techniques of physical restoration but not how to understand the moral problems which confront them and their patients. Should we not do so?

7

THE ROLE OF WELFARE

L. IRIS PONTING

Miss L. Iris Ponting is a Welfare Officer of the Lambeth Borough Council in London.

What is the role of Welfare in our present society? In Britain we are cared for from the cradle to the grave. The State provides for everyone; we have free medical attention, free education, old age pensions, social security benefits and unemployment allowances. Many of the problems of previous generations no longer exist and yet stress and distress exists in no small measure in society. The statistics for people suffering from nervous diseases, the suicide rate, the crime rate, alcoholism, drug addiction and venereal diseases have all risen. More people take sedatives and tranquilizers in the hope of coping with the stress of everyday living.

People are Individuals

One of the facts too often overlooked today is that we are all individuals; each one of us is a unique person, so we cannot thrive on preconceived ideas of set groups. We are all subjected to high pressure salesmanship which emphasise material well-being. We are made aware through mass media of dramatic news from all parts of the world as soon as it happens, but it is rare that the ordinary and everyday events of our own lives hit the headlines. Increasingly we are living in a society where everything is more vast and more impersonal. In a study I carried out amongst young people, nearly all those living in large blocks of flats did not think of their dwelling places as homes, but only as boxes, somewhere to eat and to sleep. Those who went to very large schools did not feel that they were part of them, but only members of small groups. The little shop where one was known and welcomed has gone to make way for the super-market; business mergers are making the places where people work into ever larger organizations. Many feel that they have very little say in the running of their own lives, and this often leads to frustration and boredom. Yet we are above all individuals, and each of us is seeking for and working out his place in life. Is it surprising if someone who has lost, or never had, the security of a happy family back-ground, may sometimes look to artificial stimuli to assist in the problem of living? Life too for some is strained by a momentum in living for which they were not designed.

Unfortunately for many religion is not a reality. They have not known or grown up with it; it has only been a 'lesson' learned at school. It seems only too easy to drift if we have no sense of purpose or aim, if we do not make the effort to reason why we are here and ask ourselves whither we are going. The happiness of human beings is bound up in the objective of something to live for, a need for security and a feeling of belonging.

Personal Problems

Recently I was sitting on a park bench with an alcoholic, when she suddenly said, 'I had a nice home once, and then my child died of cancer. People were very kind, but they all had their own lives to lead. Work helped, but it was the loneliness, not having anybody who belonged to me, any-body to plan for. One day I went into a public house and had a drink. It was just for the company, but it helped. After a while one drink was not enough. So I lost my job, and went from one job to another. I have been away in a home several times. Now I am here, destitute and glad to go with a man for the price of a drink.'

An immigrant mother I visited said to me, 'I am so glad you called. I was feeling so depressed. In my country I always had my relatives I could turn to. Here I know no-body, and with the children being small it is difficult for me to go out. It is the loneliness that gets me down.'

Another case was a young immigrant school girl who had been brought up by her grandparents and had only recently arrived in this country. Her mother was a stranger to her. She was faced with a new school and a completely new way of life. She felt unloved and unwanted so she satisfied her craving for demonstrative love in sex, with rather unfortunate results.

Nobody is ever given a perfect world to live in; this is something we have to try and make for ourselves with such attributes as we are born with or acquire during childhood. To make a success of ourselves we have to learn to shoulder responsibilities, to live with others, to give and take and to be tolerant. It is because many people are not learning this lesson either in the home or at school that so many of today's problems exist.

I was talking to a beatnik, who described her way of life. I told her about a young girl I met in the course of my work who had been a prostitute. This girl said that one day when she was sitting in a cafe she entered into conversation with another woman who was sharing the table. She was horrified to learn that the woman was only twenty-four years old, as she looked so haggard and care worn. She too was a prostitute. The sight of this woman appalled the young girl, so when she returned to her room, she looked in the glass and thought to herself that she still had her looks, was not known to the police, and that the way was still open to her to return home and take a job. 'I wonder if you can appreciate,' she said, 'what it is like to earn in a week what you have been previously paid in one night, and to have to work regular office hours?' She still keeps away from the places where she knows she may meet other prostitutes, in case she should weaken and return to her old life. The young beatnik I was talking to got up, held out her hand, and said with emotion, 'I have not yet solved my own problems, but your story has helped.'

Some of the young people whom I interview talk about the inequalities which still exist in our society. I always answer that working in a hospital one cannot help but realize that there is *no* equality in painful illness or death.

One of the failures of our age is in personal relationships. There is often a very real lack of communication, and unfortunately for many this is also true of home life. This sometimes makes it easier for patients to discuss their problems with somebody outside the family circle. There are others who, owing to their way of life, find it almost impossible to communicate even with people at hospital. One nineteen year old was completely apathetic. I asked her if nothing gave her pleasure or interested her, and she said, 'No, I've done it all, haven't I?' 'All' included prostitution, alcohol, and drug taking.

A sojourn in hospital can be a traumatic experience for both patient and relative. Frequently a patient finds courage to adjust to his disability. For the relative, it may mean suddenly having to face problems which alter his whole way of life. Recently I was talking to a widower, who described to me what happened on the night he learnt that his wife was dying. He said, 'I came away from hospital in a daze and just walked and walked. Then I felt I would like to talk to somebody before I returned to an empty home. I ran over in my mind the list of people I could telephone, and I pictured them answering, and feared I would detect in their voices a slight urgency to return to an interesting television programme or some other home pleasure. So I made my way home, knowing that I was now on my own. At times, even for those with faith, God's Will is not easy to accept and understand, yet by accepting it one is given peace of mind.' This story of solitude brings home the result of lack of neighbourliness. No longer do we know who lives next door; a barrier has grown up, which excludes us from everything except conversational platitudes. Seldom do we feel we can talk of our troubles to others, however great may be the need. This generation may have all the material needs met, but human compassion is sadly lacking.

The Aim of Welfare

The welfare services form a countrywide network in every field of human suffering, and it would be impossible to enumerate all the excellent work which is being done. However the types and kinds of problems are constantly changing, and there is still a great deal that needs to be done. Some problems are difficult to solve owing to changes in the family pattern and our present stringent financial situation; for example the right type of housing, and sufficient domestic help for the aged, the disabled and the chronically sick are still sadly inadequate.

At the beginning of this account I posed the question, 'What is the role of Welfare?' It is not only to help people with their problems, to make known to them all the facilities which are available. There is also a need for someone with whom you can talk over an emotional problem, someone who will listen sympathetically. The ideal is to give a personal service in a world which is becoming increasingly impersonal.

8

DRAMA AS A THERAPEUTIC FORCE

Rev. ALAN THORNHILL, M.A.

*The Rev Alan Thornhill, once Chaplain of Hertford
College, Oxford, has become a playwright, and is
associated especially with the Westminster Theatre
in the West End of London.*

What do we expect of the Theatre?

You may wonder what in the name of Hippocrates the
theatre has to do with therapy. 'Can't we just be left in
peace,' I can almost hear someone say, 'to go to an
occasional show, without having to ask if it's good for us?'
In fact I have vivid memories of Mr R. V. Cooke, the warm-
hearted and out-spoken President of the B.M.A., saying to
me just before he took the chair when I first gave a talk on
the subject, 'I can't imagine for the life of me what you are
going to talk about, but I'm looking forward to it enormously.'

The truth is, of course, that if we are thinking about a
healthy society, there are few aspects of the subject more
important than entertainment. In fact it could be argued
that art and entertainment, in all their various forms, may
do more to affect the health of society, either for good or
ill, than religion and politics put together. I do not say that
this ought to be so, but it is quite possible that it is.

'I knew a very wise man,' wrote Andrew Fletcher of
Saltoun nearly 300 years ago, 'who believed that if a man
were permitted to make all the ballads, he need not care
who should make the laws of a nation'. If that wise man
had lived in the days of films, TV programmes, subsidised
theatre, pop singers and the rest, he might have felt ten
times more strongly the effect of 'entertainment' on the life
and character of the nation. And although I am confining

myself to only one small section of the whole field of entertainment – namely the 'live' theatre – it is nevertheless a part
that has a very great influence on the rest. 'For this writing
of plays', said Bernard Shaw, 'is a great matter, forming as
it does the minds and affections of men in such sort that
whatsoever they see done on the stage, they will presently
be doing in earnest in the world which is but a larger stage.'

What do we expect when we go the theatre? Entertainment – relaxation – excitement – escape? Or, if we are
more demanding, we may look for artistic satisfaction, some
touch of beauty, some moment of truth, some fresh insight
into life and the kind of creatures that we really are. Often,
I am afraid, we find none of these things – only perhaps
boredom, frustration, exasperation or a general sense of
not having got our money's worth.

Perhaps there is something beyond what I have mentioned
to be found in the theatre. Do we expect anything to
happen when we go to a play? After all 'Happenings', a
word greatly loved by the *avant garde,* are of the essence of
drama. Aristotle's famous definition of Tragedy is 'the imitation of an action' – not just words or emotion, but action.
In drama things are not just said, they happen.

What happens to the Audience?
The known history of drama goes back as far as the fourth
millenium B.C. Certain texts inscribed on the interior walls
of pyramids and tombs are clearly dramatic in form with
directions for action and indications of various characters
speaking. We have the full text of one play dating from
the second millenium B.C.; there are forty-six scenes with
full stage directions, lists of props and *dramatis personae.*
All these ancient pieces of theatre are religious, one might
say ritualistic, in nature. They are to be performed on special
occasions such as at the death of the king. The newly appointed king is required himself to play the leading part
and, with the help of the audience, i.e. the whole populace,
actually to fight for his throne against all rivals and forces
of evil!

There is at least one example of a medicinal drama, whose
purpose is magical or faith healing. It is the story of the

goddess Isis whose child Horus has been bitten by a scorpion and involves artificial respiration and a magical cure.

In all this ancient Egyptian theatre, and in ancient Greece too, what is done by and what happens to the audience seems to be just as important and just as much part of the drama as anything that happens 'on the stage'.

It is still the playwright's hope and dream that the drama will in some sense take place in front of as well as behind the floodlights. He is always looking for those golden moments, rare and often unaccountable, when the barrier between stage and spectators melts away and something is born and lives and grows in the imagination and experience of actors and audience together. A play cannot truly be said to exist until it has been experienced in performance before an audience, because every play is partly the creation of its audience as they fill out in their imaginations what they see and hear from the stage. 'The music of humanity,' said *The Times* dramatic critic in an unusually human review, 'that rare and precious sound in the Theatre, steals over the house.'

One of the most encouraging moments that I as a playwright have ever known in the theatre was during the first production of my first play. It took place in a tiny barn theatre in the country, where the audience and the actors were only a few feet apart. The scene was in the kitchen of a labour leader's home during a tense and bitter strike. A running fire of argument and accusation between the labour leader and his wife went back and forth across the breakfast table over the head of their small son, as he sat eating his cornflakes between them. It was at that point that I realised that I was sitting in the audience just behind an actual labour leader, who had come out from the big city with his wife to see the play. I could see that both of them were lost in rapt attention. The wife especially was leaning forward following every line of dialogue as if it was her own. Suddenly, in the scene, there was an unexpected knock on the door. The wife in the audience shouted, 'Come in'. The laughter that followed interrupted the play, but it was music in the ear of the author. He knew that at any rate for one person the magic of the theatre had worked. Something had 'happened'.

I have sometimes thought since that the object of the whole business of theatre is that somebody present should say, 'Come in' – to a thought, an emotion, a shock or a realisation, never experienced in that particular way before. But, if that is so, the responsibility of those who engage in theatre is very great. For we can say, 'Come in' to what is true or to what is false, to something healing or to something hurtful, to spiritual vitamins or to deadly poison.

For the classical description of drama as a therapeutic force we turn again to Aristotle. 'A tragedy', he says, 'is the imitation of an action ... with incidents arousing pity and fear wherewith to accomplish a catharsis of such emotions.' So Aristotle, considering the Greek theatre of his day, regards it as a catharsis, that is to say a purifying of the audience and through the audience of society itself. Going to the theatre in those days was a serious business. You arrived early in the morning before the sun rose. You sat through the greater part of the day and watched probably three tragedies and one comedy. The audience was noisy and enthusiastic and quite capable of throwing stones at a wretched author who failed to meet with its approval. Going to the theatre was an act of worship. It was also part of the duty of a good citizen; everyone was expected to go. Even the slaves had a seat and if you were too poor to pay, the State would pay for you. In fact, at times you were liable to pay a fine if you did not go to the theatre, a practice which, as a playwright, I would wholeheartedly approve. The point is that knowing the violent and powerful and destructive passions which lie within the heart of man, the ancient Greeks regarded the theatre as a way to bring out and to purify and redirect these passions into channels that were wholesome, both for the individual and society. Through pity or compassion, men could be brought to realise the immense capabilities in man, both for greatness and for evil, and through fear, to understand the awful consequences of the kind of lives that we live and the choices that we make.

Similarly, comedy was in its different way a purifying

influence. As a professor of mine at Oxford used to say, 'Laughter is the shout of welcome with which we greet ourselves'.

One could trace this conception of the theatre down through the ages from the mystery and morality plays performed in our churches and cathedrals, right on to the dramas of social conscience in Ibsen, Galsworthy and Shaw. Bernard Shaw once described the theatre as 'A factory of thought, a prompter of conscience and elucidator of social conduct, an armoury against despair and dullness, and a temple of the ascent of man'.

Plays that heal the Ills of our Age

It is against this background that I would like to present my own experience of theatre as a healing force in society today. At a conference which I was attending in America ten years ago, there appeared out of the blue a great singer and actress, Muriel Smith, an American Negro. She had looked in at the conference for two days on the advice and encouragement of some friends. At that time, the racial ferment in America was beginning to boil up. The name of Little Rock was in the headlines. Muriel Smith, as a Negro artist, had always had a longing to use her gifts in some way to help her own people and her country. At the conference she saw her chance. She made a bold decision and cancelled an extremely attractive offer to play in a big film in Hollywood. She gave up a contract to sing for another season in Covent Garden. She felt that more important than any of these things was to produce some kind of play that could help to bring healing to Little Rock and all that it symbolised. Together some of us at the conference wrote a musical play called *The Crowning Experience,* based on the story of a great American Negro pioneer in education, Mary McLeod Bethune.

When the play was ready, we took it with a cast of a hundred actors representing many races, both black and white, to the city of Atlanta, the largest city in the South of the United States. Many people at that time were saying that all that was happening in Little Rock was just a picnic compared with what would follow in Atlanta. They told us that within two days we would be thrown out on our ear. But in Atlanta we found a theatre owner who responded; he was a Jew of vision and courage. He said, 'You may use my theatre as long as you can fill it, and I am going to do something that has not been done in Atlanta for a hundred years. I am going to open the doors of my theatre and let everyone come in and sit together, black and white.'

The play ran in the finest theatre in Atlanta for more than four months, and night after night all the races came in and sat and experienced it together. There was much fear in that theatre in Atlanta and there was pity too. There was also through the spirit and artistry of a woman like Muriel Smith a cathartic, a healing force. At the end of the run a leading Negro lawyer in Atlanta said, 'This city will never be the same again. There is a new spirit abroad. You can feel it in the streets, in the buses, in the shops and in the schools.' I would be the last person to suggest that all the problems of Atlanta are solved, that there is not still injustice and discrimination, and that there will never be the kind of violence there that other American cities have been seeing so tragically. But it is significant that over the years, Atlanta has made quiet and steady progress in the right direction through the combined effort of white and black alike.

Two or three years ago a historical play of mine about William Wilberforce was performed at the Westminster Theatre and then went on tour through England. The last week of its run was in the elegant eighteenth-century theatre in Bath. At one of the performances, there came three militant, extreme Left-wing, dockers' leaders from Bristol, who had just been leading an unofficial strike which had held up the whole Port of Bristol for several weeks and which cost a million pounds. A historical play in Bath did not seem the most likely setting in which to interest or influence men such as these. Indeed, one of them had never in his life seen a live stage play before. But something about the courage and humanity of Wilberforce gripped Jack Carroll, the dockers' leader, in the theatre that night. 'That fellow Wilberforce,' he said, 'had the guts to challenge his own crowd, the Establishment of the day, and give them hell for the fat profits they were making out of human flesh and blood. He fought them in and out of Parliament for thirty years and he won.' Carroll returned to Bristol, first to make peace within his own home, which was on the point of breaking up. Then he went to the leaders of his Union from whom he had been alienated, and found a working basis with them. One of them, Ron Nethercott, head of the Transport and General Workers Union in the area, says, 'Jack Carroll has changed very much. Formerly he would get in a shouting match and not listen to you. At the end of an hour I'd have got so bloody annoyed I wouldn't have known what he was talking about.' Together they tackled Management and began to pioneer new conditions and practices and above all a new spirit in the Port of Bristol. George Edney, General Manager of the Port of Bristol Authority, describes the change in Carroll and his friends as 'one of the reasons we have had so little trouble in the Port of Bristol since decasualisation'. Not only did Bristol keep open during the dock strikes of 1967–8, but Carroll's influence was felt in other British ports. In 1968, too, he took unpaid leave to visit the docks of India, where he and others were instrumental in resolving an inter-union dispute that was holding up the unloading of grain needed to relieve famine in Bihar. Remarkable action for any former trouble-maker to take, and it all began in a theatre.

A Theatre that restores Faith

The Westminster Theatre where I am proud to work – it was by the way, originally a Church and a proprietary Chapel – was bought by its present trustees after the Second World War as a memorial to the men of Moral Re-Armament who gave their lives. Its aim is to produce plays that not only entertain but help to create that kind of world which those men died to bring. It is a commercial theatre which treats its actors well, seeks to give its audiences their money's worth, and pays its way without subsidy. But beyond all that, it aims to bring about the kind of 'Happening' that will affect the health and sanity, both of the individuals who go there, and of society.

Actors who work at the Westminster are sometimes surprised at the kind of fan mail they receive. Letters come in, not only admiring a particular person or performance, but describing in specific terms the after-effects of the play. A group of nurses from a London hospital who attended a play together wrote to thank the leading lady for a new spirit and a new efficiency pervading their ward. It was the result they said of their experiencing the play together. A miner's leader from the North wrote to describe the succesful efforts he and his colleagues had made to keep their pit open and their village employed in face of threatened closure by the authorities. It was the play that had given him the added incentive to fight the battle. An industrial nurse writes with a detailed account of improvement in one of her patients as a results of a visit to the theatre. 'Could it be,' she adds, 'that a visit to a theatre can inspire, can raise the level of one's thinking and show things in perspective? Like climbing to the top of a mountain and viewing the landscape and then deciding to go home by a better way?'

Many people today do not understand this conception of theatre. The Greeks I think would have, and so would the Medieval Church. There is an old newspaper saying, 'Anything positive is propaganda, anything negative is news', and there is a theatrical version of that sentiment which says, 'Anything faith-giving is preaching, anything faith-destroying is art'. But perhaps the Westminster Theatre is pointing a trend of the future. As Peter Howard, who did so much to pioneer it, said, 'I want to see the British theatre once more play its part in restoring honour to homes, unity between colours and classes, and to all men faith in God'.

9

THE CARING COMMUNITY

R. A. LAMBOURNE, B.D., M.B., CH.B., D.P.M.

Dr Lambourne combines the roles of psychiatrist and theologian. He is Lecturer in Pastoral Studies at the University of Birmingham and Clinical Assistant to the Rubery Hill Hospital, Birmingham. He is the author of Community, Church and Healing.

During the last thirty years an increasing interest has been shown by professionals working in the medical and social services in the part which the 'caring community' can play in assisting in their work. This growing interest reverses a pre-war tendency amongst social reformers, very many of whom felt that with technological progress and the coming of the welfare state voluntary work for the sick not only could but should disappear. These reformers felt that voluntary caring, and indeed any caring or healing outside the organised professional services, was an unhappy relic of an unjust society which patched up its inadequate provisions by second rate substitutes in the shape of voluntary work. It was considered that such work was not only second rate but also covered up deficiencies and delayed reform. It was further supposed that every problem of sickness would sooner or later be so objectified that there would be a professional remedial organisation that would solve it in the same style as was already largely successful in overcoming conditions like acute appendicitis.

There has been a reaction from these positions and now much more is heard about 'community care' and 'the caring community'. Clear distinctions are now made between 'community care' as the best policy and 'community care' as a second best policy or as a strategy for avoiding the expense of a first rate service. 'Community care' is now regarded as a genuine option and the part which friends and relatives play in maintaining the health of the nation receives some attention and a little of the research it deserves. In geriatrics, for example, it is generally acknowledged that sheer weight of numbers makes a total non-domestic service prohibitive in cost and personnel. But, more important to our case, it is also accepted that even if such a service were practicable it would not be ideal for the elderly, many of whom are happier and more useful at home.

This first concept of 'the caring community' as care by relatives and friends is, then, widely known and widely acceptable. So is a second concept, in which stress is laid upon the measures taken by a local statutory body, in Britain the Local Authority, to supplement the other medical services, especially by the employment of professionals in the medical and social service fields. However, these two ideas of 'the caring community' have often been reached without much thought. It will here be argued that they fall short of the full concept of 'the caring community' and that whilst representing much good they are too weak to modify certain better entrenched ideas which are antagonistic to their prosperity. Therefore a third, more radical and stronger concept of the meaning of 'a caring community' will be discussed below, which if it became influential would enable the other two understandings to prosper.

Voluntary Help

The first concept of 'the caring community' is essentially the idea of a comparatively well person helping a comparatively ill person. It is a one-to-one relationship. The caring usually consists of fairly distinctive acts which may constitute the whole of the relationship of the two people, and sometimes such acts may be organised and channelled through special associations. They thereby differ from those caring activities, of which a mother's care is a good example, where the acts so blend into personal relationships that they are seen as functions of that relationship. Though not usually thought of as professional, they are similar to professional work in that the caring act is relatively isolated from other relationships and is recognised as such by both parties, as when volunteers visit the sick in hospitals or run Telephone Samaritans. In this category come the activities of many thousands of people who do sick visiting, run car clubs for the disabled, deliver 'meals on wheels', mind children, do night watching, man ambulances, and give many other services. They range from kind deeds within the normal give and take of family life, of neighbours, or of work colleagues, to very specialised work like that done by those who are trained to assist the Probation Officers.

The motivation and mobilisation of such men and women to constitute a caring community follows a long and strong religious tradition which has Judaeo-Christian roots in the Western world. As an activity of the local Christian congregation it continues Christ's healing ministry, demonstrating the power of thoughtful love to heal, and the will of God that all men should be made whole.

This then is the first concept of 'the caring community'. It is one of voluntary help directed to meet special needs rather in the way the professional does it but usually not demanding so much skill.

This last statement about skill may however become less true with the passage of years, for as we move towards a more highly educated and leisurely community many more volunteers are being trained to professional standards. In one hospital in the U.S.A., the Lutheran General, Chicago, the voluntary help given includes manning of enquiry desks, running catering facilities and doing the electro-cardiographs. Several hospitals in this country are now employing a full time member of staff to co-ordinate and train the voluntary workers. One effect of this type of trained caring community work is that it brings the layman into closer touch with the professional. However, whether it thereby encourages an increasingly distinctive lay contribution is questionable. For one of the side effects of being trained by the professional is increasing identification with him and adoption of the professional viewpoint rather than that of the patients and relatives. Sometimes one needs to be concerned but detached in order to discern the truth, and training can make detachment difficult.

The first concept of the caring community involving, as it

does, unremunerated work, depends partly upon a belief that an act of concern and love is good in itself. Of course this pure charity is held in the earthen vessel of mutual aid systems which every group and every society operates, and it is regulated in a very sophisticated way by social custom. However, the act of pure charity does occur without expectation of any recompense, not even the goodwill or gratitude of the recipient or the approval of society. Such acts demonstrate a belief in human qualities which, whilst held by many besides theists, does seem to many people to be especially reasonable for the theist. Certainly such acts are our defence against cynicism. They are not merely the ground on which good citizenship is built but the means of renewal in man of his own faith, hope and love.

The Local Authority's Contribution

The second concept of the caring community is defined not by its voluntary nature but by its local as distinct from its national origin and support. This leads in Britain to the idea of statutory work done by the Local Authority as distinct from a much larger authority such as the state. In this concept of the caring community, often under the title of 'community care', the expectation of individual unpaid acts of concern is often less, but the individual's expectation that 'they should do something' is increased, and 'they' are paid officers of the Local Authority. These same representatives of the caring community often observe that 'the community couldn't care less' thereby highlighting their sense that the first concept of the caring community described above is vital to their work within the second concept.

At the back of this confusion may be the belief that Local Authority services automatically depend more upon the interest and support of people for one another than services provided by a national authority. Unfortunately, such interest and support is not always forthcoming, and an employee of a Local Authority visiting a patient or client in his home may find that people in the client's neighbourhood have no more sense of responsibility to assist him than they would if the attempt to help was taking place ten miles away in a large District Hospital. Indeed these neighbours may see the

Local Authority's provision of a paid worker as evidence that voluntary care of each other is unnecessary and outmoded, and so with an easy conscience they may turn aside from their neighbour's distress. Thus is set one of the main problems of our day, in which the welfare state by a gradual replacement of old implicit mutual aid structures may erode that basic minimum of mutual concern and local political responsibility which a healthy society needs. It may thus produce a community of low morale, which creates a fresh crop of human needs, which leads to fresh statutory provision, and so on in a vicious circle.

Individual special needs are relatively easily definable and measured, and therefore easily provoke public concern. The same cannot be said of the slow decline in local community health measured not only by such criteria as for instance hospital admissions, but also in more truly corporate terms such as the level of mutual concern shown by personal acts, the level of responsible political action to improve the neighbourhood, and the general level of hope and belief in a dignified human life. An Aberfan produces emergency measures, but a gradual landslide in a local community's morale which kills more bodies and more spirits produces no such sense of urgency. In the world of medical care an acute illness in one individual provokes greater concern than a slow community decline, despite the fact that the latter may be more ominous in terms of morbidity rates, let alone in terms of a full life.

A Wider Concept

A third concept of community care, which tends to reverse this priority, does so by examining the full context of each medical or social service. It always scrutinises carefully any proposed change in these services to enquire whether it is not only good in itself, that is within its own terms of reference, but whether it is good within a wider, communal, ecological view of a healthy society. This third concept, a truly corporate concept, of the caring community will now be discussed. It will be suggested that since it always implies the effort to define, measure and strive for medical health within the context of the overriding goal of a new society

100

and a new experience of a good life in fellowship, it lies within the main stream of the Judaeo-Christian religious tradition, but finds itself somewhat at odds with those who see the magnification of individual medical health as the goal above goals.

The model of disease and healing used by the medical profession has been changing and increasing in complexity over the last two hundred years. Nineteenth-century medicine was largely dominated by what may be called a focal-physical model. This was natural to a society accepting mechanistic models of the world and man, and to a Medicine which largely owed its emergence as a science to anatomists and histologists who naturally saw normality and defects in terms of stationary structures. The influence of the biological as distinct from the physicists' revolution was yet to be felt. So the model of disease was of a local structural blemish, and healing was its removal. This model is indeed still the dominant one, and the skill of isolating pathology and actually manually removing it still earns for the doctor the greatest praise and reward both within and outside the profession. The dramatic act of excision and removal or substitution still keeps this model of healing well to the forefront even though in fact it does poor justice to the art of the surgeon and his team for whom the actual excision may be a minor part of their task.

With the development of experimental physiology in the last century the focal model of disease began to be modified by a more systematic one, so that healing was seen less as the elimination of a bad focus in an organ of the body and much more as returning a physiological system to a state of balance which had been temporarily disturbed. The discovery of various neural and hormonal feedback mechanisms, some of which linked individual physiological systems, gradually produced a model of health and disease in which the body is considered as a whole.

Since then we have moved further to include in this holistic model first the psyche and then other persons and other forms of environment. Nowadays this new ecological model based upon biological analogies is making itself felt. This means that the individualistic model of health is now under tension with an ecological one. The logic of this is that in principle any claims for effective treatment of a particular disease are not acceptable if they are based exclusively on evidence derived from the study of treatment of a number of isolated individuals suffering from that particular disease. For if the unit of health and disease is more than an individual then measurement of presence and absence of disease must include in its view more than that individual. Of course, what is in principle true of all disorders may be of more obvious practical importance in some than others. Thus in psychiatry and infectious diseases an epidemiological approach is now orthodox.

In the developing countries we have been given striking evidence of thousands of lives being saved in hospitals from particular diseases yet with no change in local mortality figures. Faced with such figures the doctor may of course insist that it is his duty to save from immediate death each individual as he presents himself at hospital with a particular disease. He may be right, but if it seems self evidently so to anyone, it is because an individualistic model has dominated medicine. This may be connected with a particular individualistic idea of the sacredness of life and of salvation which has dominated much modern Christian thinking especially in Protestantism. However, nowadays many factors including family psychiatry, social medicine, national planning of economic development in unison with health programmes, and ethology, are all encouraging the measurement of health within the context of the total life of a people.

Some of the diseases previously seen as organic problems within an individual are now seen as the effects of stress. Such stress in its turn may be considered as a sign of stress involved in national change. If, for example, we regard drug addiction as a disease, it is surely as effective to regard it as a social disease which breaks out in persons, as to regard it as a disease of the individual. Moreover the disease which appears may be one only of many alternative signs of such stress. Consequently what looks like a phenomenal success in reducing the rate of one such class of disease may just be a success in moving the stress into another disease. It is to be hoped that in psychiatry especially a very ecological view will be taken, particularly as health programmes are mounted around crisis situations, such as bereavement. For example, to show that such and such a procedure is associated with a reduction of post-bereavement depression is not sufficient evidence on which to make that procedure a routine hygienic measure, because the procedure may have far-ranging cultural effects.

With the ecological view advocated above tension must rise between an individualistic and a corporate view of health. 'The Doctor's Dilemma' is really with us and we have to learn to live with it. It is a pity that in all the recent ethical discussions this problem has been given comparatively little attention and the theology concerned has been left almost untouched. In fact the concept of a corporate unit of health has a strong theological background. Under pressure from this theology the central credo in medicine that where an individual can be healed he must be healed takes a jolt. We must now consider this theological background of the caring community and especially the corporate element in that concept.

Salvation and Health in the Old Testament

Old Testament studies of the last fifty years have concerned themselves a good deal with understanding its Semitic and Hebraic background, and it has been emphasised that to understand the theological ideas of the Old Testament this background must be taken seriously. The social, economic, and political experiences of the Hebrew people were different from our own, and with this difference went distinctive ways of thought. Thus whilst in the Old Testament great stress is placed upon personal responsibility, this responsibility is shown by the part that particular persons play in community care, that is in God's dealings with the well-being and goodness of His people and with their deliverance. Personal righteousness is not an individual matter, for it is inseparable from the context of the Covenant of God with His people. The Old Testament uses many images of deliverance upon which models of healing and salvation can be based, but they all work within this general image of a Covenant between God and a people. This is a strongly corporate model. God's concern for the particular person is woven into His plan to deliver His people within His Covenant. Thus deliverance, and hence health and salvation for all men, is not the end result of delivering men and women one by one until arithmetical addition shows that all have been saved. Nor is the People of God, the healthy community, the saved community, a social contract whereby individuals who find themselves to be delivered join together because of their common point of view, common experiences, and common goals. On the contrary the very idea of a delivered individual in the midst of an undelivered people presents difficulties to the Hebrew thought forms of the Old Testament. To be healthy on one's own is for them a logical contradiction, since the man who is cut off from God's people is dead.

The strength of this corporality is well exemplified by the weakness of the idea of individual survival after death within the images of resurrection as they slowly develop in the Old Testament and Apocrypha. The strongest images of resurrection in the Old Testament show it occurring corporately in this world and not individually outside this world as in the popular contemporary views of heaven. Individual survival is weakly portrayed in the weakness of Sheol. Powerful resurrection is portrayed in holistic images as the People of God are resurrected to new life in fellowship and justice *together,* as in Ezekiel's vision of the resurrection of the dry bones of a people, or in Isaiah's ecological images of the whole created order coming to corporate harmony and the wolf lying down with the lamb.

Resurrection is God's gift of health together to a people who have been promised this within His Covenant. And what is this Covenant? It is to serve God *as a people.* This service of God includes the service of each other within the Covenanted people, and in the New Testament especially it becomes the corporate service of all men. Christ, representing the Covenanted people, the healthy community, demonstrates His perfection and thus the wholeness and health of the saved community by caring for others. The model of health suggested by this is that of a corporate group who are healthy in dying for others.

Health and the Christian Community

It will be seen from the Biblical evidence cited above that the popular contemporary individualistic view of health takes a double knock. First, because the final signs of health are to be judged within a wide framework of shared fellowship (as for example the sharing of scarce medical resources). Secondly, because this health is given within a caring for others which involves a sacrifice of health as the world sees it. By such criteria a man who demands perfect health for himself whilst others still lack health is both contradicting a law of neighbourliness and attempting a logical absurdity. The caring community is one which is based upon the faith that it will be given health in community when it forgets its health in the passionate (consider Christ's Passion) concern and action for others outside itself. Within the Christian tradition this is an act of faith which continues the act of faith made by Christ, who trusted that if He gave His health in giving health to others God would raise Him up. It continues too the act of faith in Christ's belief about health which was demonstrated by the early Church in their preaching of the Resurrection.

Now this is very different from the individualistic models of health which dominate our world in which the right of an individual to possess the best health for himself has been raised to the status of an idolatry. Then my health, or the health of a nation, becomes a god above gods before which every other consideration must bow. Health seems so obviously a good thing that we can pursue it unthinkingly with a sigh of relief that here is one ethic which is not situational.

However, on reflection we can see that this is dubious to say the least. We know that doctors and nurses are daily arriving from the developing countries to work for us. Yet the case of overseas medical personnel is only one easily seen example of the dangers of using the individual as the unit of health. Usually it is 'the sacredness of individual life' which is used in arguments to support such an action. But those who claim Christian support for this idea of the sacredness of individual life do so by disregarding a mainstream in the theology of the Bible. Life as a biological phenomenon, measured for example by longevity, has nothing sacred about it. It is first of all fellowship and love between man and man, and man and God which are sacred. They are sacred in the sense that they represent God's undefeatable goal for His creation, and also partake of a quality of His own life. Only within this context can my neighbour's health or my own health be safely spoke of as sacred. Outside it the concept has Biblical condemnation and not support. The pursuit of health for myself or for my group as an unconditional and unquestionable right is demonic.

The concept of the caring community is not then an idea supporting an important but peripheral adjunct to modern medicine but a revolutionary idea which raises great tensions within the accepted ways of thought and practice in the medical profession and health services. The problems which arise in medical ethics when the doctor's public responsibilities conflict with the principle of the rights of the individual patient are just one small example. The intrusion of value judgements, including the social value of one individual against another, into clinical judgements about who will be selected for benefit from scarce resources – say renal dialysis – is another. Priorities in selecting 'at risk' groups for national health planning is a third.

The Biblical concept of the caring community puts an emphasis on a social context and estimation of health. This is challenge enough. But the emphasis which springs from the identification of Christ with the caring community, and of Christ with the Suffering Servant, means that within the caring community whilst pain and discomfort remain an unqualified evil they are yet part of man's movement towards health and wholeness and as such are within God's providence. Because Christ, the Man for Others, is shown as *perfect yet suffering* within that service the perfect caring community is *perfect yet suffering*. This has its dangers; it easily leads to masochism or to telling other people that they must suffer because it is God's will. Yet, though the idea has a mixed history and a deservedly questionable reputation, without it the other idea, that a person has an absolute right not to suffer, is equally destructive. The latter has probably played a part in making that section of medicine which helps incurable people to live as whole persons be given less regard than is its due.

The corporate model of deliverance and salvation, and thus health, which we find in the Bible, is very distinct from the individualistic ideas of personal salvation which have held sway in Christian theology, especially among many Protestants in the last two hundred years. The concept of the religious life as the individual striving by himself to overcome moral faults by the sole aid of one dominant Healer is vigorously challenged by both the Old Testament understanding of the People of God and the New Testament understanding of the fellowship in Christ – the Church. It was the religious understanding of salvation as individual salvation which in its secular form shaped modern medicine as we know it today and gave it deficiencies as well as strength. If we take the individualistic religious model and for moral faults we substitute diseases, and for aid direct from God outside the social fellowship we substitute direct aid from the professional outside the society to which the patient belongs, then the medical model of today is apparent. Medical psychiatrists copied this model from surgery and internal medicine to give the one-to-one situation of analyst and patient striving to remove blocks to wholeness by therapy given outside the social context and in the privacy of the consulting room. These same psychiatrists sometimes dreamed up utopias in which individuals would be saved one by one by analysis until all the world was saved. This was an individualistic model of salvation and deliverance and health. Recent trends in psychiatry towards family and community models may thus be seen not as a new invention but a shift back towards the Biblical understanding of that caring community within which alone health is given and understood. To live as a Covenanted people in true fellowship with one another and with God is the prescription for health in the Judaeo-Christian tradition. Of such a fellowship love is both the condition and the evidence. It is within this prescription that the healing which modern medicine pursues finds its place, and outside that prescription it becomes idolatrous. In particular, love and fellowship with man and God are not recommended solely as a means to being what we would call 'healthy', but are an integral part of salvation, wholeness, God's health for man. Love and fellowship are not, for example, good only because they can be demonstrated to facilitate health by child psychologists and others, but are part of wholeness and cannot be dispensed with. This unity between love, fellowship and 'health' expressed by the diverse images of deliverance, wholeness and salvation within the Biblical tradition is re-discovered today in the concept of 'health in the caring community', which intertwines ethical and health concepts in a unity which modern separation between the medical and religious professions has undone. Such a concept intertwining love, fellowship and health is antagonistic to those who would assess the efficacy of either medical or religious interventions into society within medical or religious categories alone, but supports those who seek always to judge such interventions in a wider context.

Lay Participation

The concept of the caring community as a group of people who find health in giving health to others has another radical implication for medicine since it carries into medicine a strong *lay* element. The caring community, the people of God, are the 'laos' and every one of them is both healer and patient. Saving is then not only the responsibility of a few priests set apart to save, and healing is not just the privilege and responsibility of a few doctors set apart to heal. Rather all are involved in a common healing and learning experience. These are ideas which we find cropping up again in our own day in hospital practice and hospital research. We read, for example, that the healing efficiency of a modern hospital is linked with capacities for interpersonal communication, change, and empathy between all who work in it, so that the whole corporate body is described as a learning community. The concept of the therapeutic community hospital is essentially that of the 'laos' giving and receiving together with openness and expectation of renewal and healing. The New Testament shows every man being saved and saving others within that caring community which St Paul calls the Body of Christ. St Peter speaks of all the caring community as the Royal Priesthood in which every member has a priestly task, and not just a few special members set apart. Thus the centre for the mediation of deliverance in the early Church is shifted from a person set apart, operating in a temple set apart, to a whole people operating in the places where they live and work.

The concept of the caring community when fully applied has then very radical implications. It represents a shift from individualism to inter-personalism, from lay consumption to lay participation, from hospital centre to community centre, and it blurs some of the sharper distinctions of role between sick and healthy, professional and lay, giver and receiver. It calls to mind the democratic community of the first days of the Christian church after Pentecost and the ideas of 'participation' and 'involvement' which are so emotive in Western European countries today. These ideas are really radical and they imply a whole restructuring of the health services and of education for it. For example, if we take them seriously then we cannot educate medical students in hospitals and theological students in theological colleges and then give them the option of a few weeks' experience in the community and a lecture or two on community services and how to work together. With almost all their experience in hospital they will already have inherited the dominant ways of seeing sickness and health from the point of view of the special person in a special place. Instead their central attitudes should be formed when they are in the formative years of medical education by the major part of their training being given whilst working in an interdisciplinary group of laity including various kinds of professionals. Note that the professional is properly included in the laity since these are not defined by being non-professionals but by their consciousness of themselves as being a living people by virtue of their involvement in bringing health to all. This consciousness is the grounds of their con-fession which includes profession. Within their corporate confession, divisions of labour and specialisation lead to the recognition of persons with very special skills. However, such persons are

not defined as professionals by being set apart from the
laity but by being set within the laity, within the caring
community. This reminds us of the Pauline model described
in I Cor 12. This point about the relation of special skills
in a lay movement is very important because advocates of a
lay theology or a lay medicine are often accused of naivety
for allegedly supposing that very complex tasks can be done
without the help of special skills. But 'lay' is not the opposite to 'professional' any more than being an amateur essentially means being less skilled than a professional. Until
we think about these things we do not realise how medicine and theology dominated by 'professionals' subtly produce damaging distortions of ideas of 'amateur', 'lay', 'professional' and 'caring community'.

Creating the Caring Community

The basic idea which has to be given expression today, as it
was after Pentecost, is that of a number of people together
seeking to discover within themselves and in the world a new
life together, a new wholeness, a new community. Thus
the early Christians discovered a new concept of wholeness and health, proclaimed it, and began to work out its
daily implications, all in one life together. The religious
revelation, the caring, the new understanding of the healthy
and whole life and its reaching and teaching was for the
Pentecostal community *one* activity, one common life. This
is the strong concept of the caring community today.

Of course such a community soon runs into practical
difficulties in our present complex and pluralistic world. A
highly organised and diversified welfare state seems to make
impossible a local corporate participation in the health services. Thus those people who are not full time members of
one particular service or agency often find that the best
they can do is fill in gaps left by the 'real' experts. However,
if a principle is really believed in, existing structures can
be changed bit by bit in the right direction by those prepared
to master the details of the structures and work to change
them over several decades. For example such ideas as the
unification of medical and social services in a particular
region, the subject of recent Government white papers,

might, if it led to real local co-operation, lead to services which are a little less resistant to the working of a caring community. Again, some recent experiments in community associations seem to encourage the kind of participating communalism which the concept of the caring community involves. In these the neighbourhood seeks to decide for itself what are the strengths and weaknesses of its area and to take action to implement its findings.

The skill, the faith and the information required for such a community caring are not acquired in a day. Where will they be found? One general source must surely come from the idea of educating for the caring community in the schools. Thus local situations might not merely provide outlets for sixth form voluntary work but the very facts from which education begins. The needs of the world might set an agenda for schools just as they should for medicine and the church. In such tasks the dispersed church and the dispersed religious person will be involved. Is there any special place for the gathered church?

Cells of people gathered together to learn to be the caring community and two or three gathered together in God's name, are really the same thing if both 'caring' and 'God' are truthfully defined. Within such self-conscious groups training may begin by their members discovering personal skills and social machinery for helping each other in the various crisis and growth points which any group of people individually and corporately experience. Sick visiting, seeking and giving of counsel, financial aid, baby sitting, radical differences of opinion, prayer, correction of injustice are all part of this. The point is that the corporate, or group, or congregational context of such activities leads to skill being gained in community care. This community training complements the individual pastoral, medical or social work care which is the present strength of the Church in the West. Such learning must not of course be perpetually confined to internal mutual caring but must be transferred out of the gathered church context into the world as a whole. Thereby what is learned from others outside can be transferred back into the gathered church as a source of insight and skill and revelation. The end result of this approach will be a gradually increasing body of knowledge, and an increasing number of groups of people mature in its application, which can balance the present overriding strength of centralised caring of which hospital based medicine is the most distinguished representative. Eventually we shall have schools of medicine based upon the caring community concept in which corporate and inter-professional co-operation will be the rule instead of the exception. Then, what look like trivial and optional community activities will be seen to have been the precursors of a great shift in medical education and medical practice. There seems no other way of balancing the present main thrust of medicine which is still directed towards overcoming defined lesions, of which effort the recent marvellous advances in transplant operations are the supreme example.

Recently the newspapers report the new Professor of Child Health at King's College, London as saying, 'Dealing with organic disease is reasonably clear cut nowadays. The frustrations come from trying to solve the problems of, say, a toddler who is not talking because he is rarely spoken to because there is only an unqualified child minder.' And again, 'You can expect more professors of transplants than paediatrics, it's that sort of world now'. But the Professor does not say that it has been that sort of world in medicine for a century now and that it is the inevitable outcome of hospital centred practice. Structures affect concepts and only a caring community structure can cultivate concepts which can balance in potency and authority those of the hospital.

To conclude, the Christian is not concerned to allege that only Christians or religious people can have the vision and the unselfishness to participate in a caring community. Far from it. However, for them Christ who was at one and the same time a unique and single person, Jesus the son of Mary, and also the representative of the Covenanted People of God, is both the example and the hope of the caring community. To put one's trust in such a flimsy idea, and such a weak reality as at present the caring community presents, and to believe that fellowship and justice are as essential to healing as the knife and the needle, *is* an act of faith. However, it is for the Christian an act of faith which identifies a man with Christ, for it was Christ who first trusted that love operating in community care through precise and non-sentimental actions would defeat disease and all other forms of evil. The Gospel tells us this and proclaims that He was not mistaken.

Further reading

G. CAPLAN: 'An Approach to Community Mental Health' (Tavistock, 1961).

R. DUBOS: 'Man Adapting' (Yale University Press, 1965).

P. L. GARLICK: 'The Wholeness of Man' (Highway Press, 1960).

M. KING (Ed.): 'Medical Care in Developing Countries' (Oxford University Press, 1966).

R. A. LAMBOURNE: 'Community, Church and Healing' (Darton, Longman and Todd, 1963).

H. A. MESS: 'Voluntary Social Service and the State' (Kegan Paul, 1948).

W. J. PHYTHIAN-ADAMS: 'The Call of Israel' (Oxford University Press, 1964).

R. EVANS: 'Standards for Morale' (N.P.H.T. Oxford University Press, 1963).

R. P. SHEDD: 'Man in Community' (Epworth, 1958).

WORLD COUNCIL OF CHURCHES: 'Health, Medical–Theological Perspectives' (Geneva, 1967).

10

A SOCIAL LABORATORY

ERNEST CLAXTON,

M.B., B.S., M.R.C.S., L.R.C.P., D.T.M. & H.

Dr Claxton is at the present time Honorary Medical Adviser to the Asia Plateau Centre for Moral Re-Armament, Panchgani, Maharashtra, India.

The Asia Plateau Centre

A laboratory need not necessarily be in a building: in the social sciences experiments usually take place in the field. From these can be learned lessons for the understanding and promotion of health. Notable examples are the Papworth village settlement for chronic T.B. cases, the silicosis investigation in South Wales, and the work on rehabilitation in the motor industry by L. W. Plewes at Luton. The settings for such enquiries may be looked upon as social laboratories. So too in the wider sense can such experiments as Mahatma Gandhi's model village of Sevagram, where an effort was made to work out a pattern of life that could be applied throughout India.

Even broader in its scope is the Asia Plateau Centre recently started by Rajmohan Gandhi, the Mahatma's grandson. It is situated at Panchgani, 4,300 feet up in the Western Ghats, 60 miles from Poona and 120 miles south of Bombay. It is a conference and residential centre, which when completed will have accommodation for 650 people.

At Asia Plateau there is a nucleus of people of different nationalities, classes and religions, who believe that the problems of India and Asia can be solved, even the ancient intractable problems of poverty and corruption. Their aim is to undergird the plans of governments, aid organisations and others by dealing with that often neglected factor, human nature.

A Social Laboratory

On the one hand there are conferences, planning with politicians and statesmen, the mounting of campaigns in different parts – all the activities necessary to reach a nation and a continent. On the other there is the ever-changing community at the Centre itself, where a new pattern of life is, as it were, on show. Moreover this pattern is spreading to the area around Panchgani.

Encounter with Rajmohan Gandhi

Before writing in more detail about Panchgani, I must explain how I became associated with it. In 1967, after twenty-two years, I retired from my career on the staff of the British Medical Association. I had been looking forward to my retirement, not because I did not enjoy the work and its outreach, but because at the age of sixty-seven it is normal after a busy job to be free from routine duties and enjoy a more leisurely life. In April of that year I met Rajmohan Gandhi, who since 1964 has been engaged to bring a 'revolution of national character' to India. He had come to Europe with a diverse yet united group of sixty young Indians, among them Brahmin and Harijan, poor and rich, Parsi, Sikh, Muslim, Christian, Buddhist and Hindu. They had written and produced a musical revue entitled 'India Arise', which they had shown to large audiences in many Asian and European countries. This they described as an 'expression of a new spirit rising in a nation'. It depicted India as it is, with all its colour and variety, its paradoxes of backwardness and progress, and contrasted it with what it can become through unselfish people devoted to bringing a solution to its problems and making the country a pattern for Asia. A great vision, I thought, but there is a mighty long way to go before such an attractive dream can be turned into reality. The very vastness of the task made it seem insurmountable. Mr Gandhi, however, is a man of faith besides having a realistic attitude to the difficulties of what he has taken on. Typical of his assessments is the following statement: 'Even a consortium of the world's cleverest leaders could not on their own, even if they had free rein, solve the problems of a country like India. They

115

would need God and they would need a new spirit in their relationship with one another.'

On another occasion he said: 'Our problem is our callousness and indifference. We just do not care for one another', yet he was also able to say: 'I am not ashamed to love India. There is gold in the hearts and minds of our people, and if it is mined it will enrich the world.'

Mr Gandhi has a practical programme for achieving his aims, as well as a force of people working with him. He is editor-in-chief of *Himmat*, a widely read weekly paper with lively and constructive comment on world issues. He also reaches the masses through films, plays and literature. One of his chief moves, of course, is the establishment of the Asia Plateau Centre where assemblies and conferences can be held. People come to it from all parts of India and from many other countries.

He has asked for 'a million people from Europe to come to Asia in the next years and decades to teach us your technical skills and, more important, to give us your heart-power, your tradition of service, your tradition of care and of faith. If I may put it so, we need from Europe the spirit of Christ, His love and His forgiveness.' He invited me and others to join him in the venture, indicating that although Britain had relinquished ties and commitments in Asia, there are still millions who look to her for leadership.

Visit to the Asia Plateau Centre

I arrived in time for the opening of the first residential block at Panchgani. Already practical results were being achieved. Old feuds were being resolved, new policies emerging and communities becoming integrated. For instance, there were two student leaders who had promoted riots, but for opposite political reasons. They found themselves sharing the same room – one would have expected a fight! – but independently each found something new, something bigger than his factional viewpoint. They learned to work together and to give constructive leadership. Another case was of an official who had been helping himself to earthquake relief funds, and selling the beds and blankets provided for victims, on the black market. He decided that to help answer corruption he must start with himself and make restitution.

Though these were still early days, major Indian and Asian issues were already being affected. New hope for Assam was beginning to emerge through leaders from that state attending conferences at Panchgani, and I shall mention later one small part of this continuing action. Reconciliations between Tamils and Sinhalese in Ceylon have also been brought about through a campaign mounted from Asia Plateau.

Medicine's Role

With the evidence of change in people and of a far-reaching programme before my eyes I began to see in a new way how Medicine could have its share in the building of the new society. It was clear to me that there was an essential part for my profession to play in this whole endeavour.

First, a medical treatment unit was needed in the Centre to deal with casual illness amongst people attending the conferences and working on the site. By caring for the health of those who are undertaking this great task, the medical profession would be making a major contribution to the whole advance.

Secondly, there was a need to improve health in the villages around Panchgani. The ideas spreading from Panchgani have in any case a positive effect on health. The application of absolute moral standards produces cleanliness in dwellings, in food and water, and consequently reduces the incidence of intestinal diseases. By dealing with the emotions of fear, resentment, bitterness, greed and jealousy, psychosomatic disorders are checked. If all this can be reinforced by professional medical advice and help, the advantages are obvious.

Thirdly, I would hope to see the medical profession adopt the ideals of Panchgani in its education and practice. I have discussed this with Deans of medical colleges, with professors and with medical practitioners. So far as the general proposition that preventive and social medicine is of major importance goes, there is no disagreement, but they are up against lifelong and age-old customs and habits.

While much can be done by improvement in sanitation, by inoculation and so on, unless you deal with human nature, you can never overcome the bulk of ill-health. At Panchgani, that is what we do.

Leading on from this is a hope I have long nourished of a further step, because in bringing a cure to divisive forces in individuals, one is also laying the foundation of a cure for those same forces in nations. The drift of the world towards war may then be halted, and Medicine, which does not otherwise appear to have any strategy for it, would be fulfilling one of the World Medical Association's aims, namely the promotion of world peace.

With all these considerations in mind I felt that I should offer to take responsibility for the medical and health aspect of the Asia Plateau Centre. I wrote home to my wife to tell her about it, and remarkably enough she got my letter the very day after she had had a strong impulse to find some new and effective form of service. As her health like mine is good, and she shares my determination to help to bring about a moral renaissance, we decided to take on the task together. First I had to return to England to raise funds and buy equipment for the project, because Panchgani depends on voluntary gifts and was already stretched to the limit financially. This took me about a year, and we finally sailed for India in November, 1968.

The medical unit at the Asia Plateau Centre has now been established at one end of the first floor of a new residential block. We have a waiting room, consulting room and surgery, and can use the adjoining bedrooms when necessary. At the opening on 25 February 1969, we had a number of doctors and nurses from round about, and the Chairman of the local branch of the Indian Medical Association performed the ceremony of cutting a bandage stretched across the passage. After inspecting the unit we all adjourned to a meeting where we told our visitors of our philosophy and what we sought to do for India. One of them wants to go with us into the villages with our message.

The health of the community we look after has been surprisingly good. By attention to the water supply and the conditions in the kitchen we have largely avoided the gastro-intestinal complaints that are so prevalent generally. It has been a terrible fight, but we are winning it. Amongst other things it has meant teaching the workers that worrying about flies and clean hands is not a European fad, but has a logical basis. After talking to them about germs, insects and so forth, we asked who would co-operate with us in defeating their harmful effects. Every hand went up.

Other Practical Activities

There are many practical activities at Panchgani. There is the building of the Centre itself; a farm where a pedigree Jersey herd is being raised, where eggs and crops are produced; the laying out and cultivation of the land to make an attractive garden; and a little school where the children of the workers have first lessons. Through all of these new life flows into the nation.

R. L. Shahi, a lecturer in civil engineering at Roorkee University, who supervised the construction of the second residential block at Panchgani, said: 'I used to be a very hard task master. But I have learnt here to have a greater human approach to workers. We have achieved something here that we normally miss in other works. Because of the atmosphere of care given to them, the workers felt deeply attached to this project and have seen it through as if they were achieving something of their dreams. From here they carry a new spirit wherever they go not only in terms of construction works but also of human relationships.'

With the construction workers came their children. Often the eight- or nine-year-olds were left to look after the younger ones while the parents worked. Such things are commonly taken for granted by the better-off people in India, but a high-caste girl of nineteen from Poona, Jayashree Sonalkar, began to get to know the children and to feel she must do something for them. With some of her friends she decided to start teaching them. As no building was available, they used the corner of a field.

The first day, a crowd of forty children of ages from one to thirteen turned up – far more than Jayashree, with no experience or training, had bargained for. She said:

'I had no idea how to manage these children, so I told

119

them about the two voices that speak in every heart, the good one and the bad one. We decided to throw out the bad and listen to the good one. As a result the children began to get honest about stealing sugar from home and money or sweets from shops. They began to put things right. Some of them for the first time in their lives decided to clean their teeth and wash themselves daily.

'They are learning reading, writing, simple arithmetic and some useful crafts, but the best lesson is how to distinguish between right and wrong.'

A Tale of Two Brothers

It is fascinating to watch the real-life dramas that take place daily under one's eyes. These constitute the heart of Panchgani's work, and they often involve nationally important situations. Here I would like to single out a story whose heroes have spent virtually all their lives here in the Kudal Valley. It is a story I have been able to follow throughout the whole period of my association with Panchgani, so I can tell it in some detail.

Maruthi, who is sixty-five, and Narayan, who is seventy, are two farmer brothers, who live in the village of Ambegar some ten miles and a thousand feet lower down the valley from Panchgani. They are leaders in the village where they each have a farm, but they have not always seen eye to eye. 'For the past fifteen years,' says Maruthi, 'there was a tug-of-war between my elder brother and myself.' The day the Asia Plateau Centre was opened, Maruthi came with his family to find out what it was all about. He was one of the crowd of four thousand that had come with the same purpose. He heard Rajmohan Gandhi speak of his aims for India, and was gripped by them. Two days later he came again and invited some of those staying at the Centre to visit his village. He became more intrigued and returned yet again with some of his friends and his brother to a meeting at the Centre. I watched their faces as they heard evidence from various speakers who told of change and reconciliation, and a new spirit coming to India and the world.

They were asked by the chairman whether they would like to know the secret. 'That is what we came for,' was the reply. They were invited to try the experiment of listening to the inner voice and writing down the thoughts that come. Maruthi had the simple thought, 'Ask your brother for his forgiveness for the years of bitterness and division'. He did this in front of others who knew of the long-standing quarrel. Narayan forgave him and apologised for his own part in the feud. Maruthi said, 'I was a man with electric connections but my fuses were out of order. That apology was like a new fuse wire and the bulb lit up.'

A year later I met them again and went to their homes. They had developed enormously, and the transformation was amazing. The passion in these men to change their country is very real, and they have filled villagers visiting them from other parts of India with a similar passion. Their change has meant longer and better work on their farm, co-operation together and consequently increased yields with enough food to last the year. Previously they had never bothered to cultivate all their land; now it is all in production. Narayan said, 'Maybe the Russians and the Americans will land on the moon, but if their hearts are not changed they will take their quarrels with them. We must cure the selfishness in the world to get peace.'

One practical step they had taken was to invite a visiting group of farmers from the West to come to their village to advise them and their neighbours. The peasants rapidly and extensively adopted suggestions for improving their tomato culture. A Canadian farmer in the party remarked that no Western farmer he knew would accept and apply new methods so swiftly.

These villagers also sent a message to the Indian Home Minister, Y. B. Chavan, who has his political base in this area. They told him they had ended the tug-of-war in their own family and village: would he end the tug-of-war in Delhi?

A Great Burmese Lady

As the doctor in charge at Panchgani I had the care of a remarkable Burmese lady, Daw Nyein Tha. She had been a leading educationist and the trusted friend of many Asian leaders. She had travelled through the world where many were captivated by her simple, vivid ways of expressing basic truths about human nature. When she flew to Panchgani from Ceylon, Daw Nyein Tha was already failing from advanced cancer of the pancreas. It was one of her last desires to see the Asia Plateau Centre – 'God's embassy', she called it – and to be part of its message of hope.

Amongst those at the Centre at the time were three senior political leaders from the state of Assam in India's North-East, where China broke through in 1962 and where there has been guerilla warfare. Although Christians, and members of the same party, the three men were at loggerheads. Daw Nyein Tha invited them all to her room together; they could hardly refuse a dying woman's request. 'You three,' she told them, 'have been chosen by God to bring unity to Assam, but you cannot do it unless you become united yourselves.' Reluctantly at first, they began to accept the idea, until eventually there came a dramatic moment at a meeting when, after an hour-long speech very much from the heart, one of them came down from the platform and offered his hand to the other two in reconciliation. They left Panchgani determined not only to work together as a team, but to endeavour to bring the unity so much needed between the hill and plains people of Assam. That a political settlement has been reached in Assam, and has some hope of proving a success, is due in no small measure to this and other action originating at and from Panchgani. The full story is too long to tell here, but I hope I have said enough to show something of Daw Nyein Tha's fight for men to find and fulfil their God-given destinies, as well as to indicate the kind of work for which the Asia Plateau Centre was created.

Her last days were a moving experience to live through. It fell to me to tell her what she already suspected, that she was going home to God. 'I am ready,' she said more than once, and this was no mere passive acceptance. She lived a day at a time, inspired and triumphant to the end.

The Significance of Panchgani

While the Asia Plateau Centre is part of a much wider action throughout India, and extending beyond its borders,

I have emphasised the work at and around the Centre itself because it is both fascinating and significant.

Being a place where people seek to live their lives according to God's pattern and God's standards, Panchgani is a growing point of God's Kingdom. In the atmosphere and framework it provides, a man becomes a better man, a doctor a better doctor, a nurse, a teacher or a social worker more efficient and effective. But the total result is far more than the sum of such individual changes. What one perceives is the beginnings of a changed society with different ways, different standards and different aims from those prevalent today.

If India is to become different, answers to her problems must be found at the level of life in her villages, as well as in the political and industrial spheres, and this is true of most Asian countries. Panchgani works on this level, yet it is precisely because the Centre has a wider out-reach that it achieves what it does. People who come here meet big conceptions, a national and international perspective, ideas that are valid universally. It is this that draws such a response, from villager and statesman alike.

U Nu, former Prime Minister of Burma and one of the great men of Asia, came to Panchgani shortly after his release from prison early in 1969. He said: 'The part that Panchgani can play in training the younger leadership could be quite unparalleled in the history of Asia'.

Part Three

The Nature of Man

11

LIFE, CHEMISTRY AND CONSCIOUSNESS

H. A. C. M^cKAY, M.A., D.SC.

*Dr McKay, as a research chemist, has studied some
of the philosophical implications of recent scientific
discoveries.*

The Chemistry of Life

Since the last war one of the greatest of scientific discoveries has stolen upon us almost unawares. We now possess part of the secret of life itself, in the sense of knowing an essential piece of the chemistry. This is knowledge of such a fundamental and revolutionary kind that we can expect the most extraordinary developments in the years immediately ahead, with awesome possibilities of our intervening in the processes that go on in the cells in our human bodies and of controlling the physical and mental characteristics of our children. There is a hope of far-reaching medical benefits, but with it a new and incalculable power of man over man.

The discovery concerns a group of substances known as nucleic acids, and especially the deoxyribonucleic acids – DNA's, for short. They are found in living cells. As is often the way the discovery can be traced through a series of stages, and the early stages gave little indication of what lay ultimately in store. First, DNA was broken down into simpler constitutents, which proved to be sugar, phosphate and four substances of the type known to the chemist as 'bases'. The four bases were

Adenosine – Thymine

Guanine – Cytosine

and they are designated by their initial letters, A, T, G and C.

Next it was shown that the sugar and the phosphate are strung together alternately to form long chains, and that there is a base attached to each sugar unit. A small piece of the chain is thus:

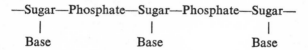

where 'Base' stands for any one of A, T, G and C.

At first it was thought that the four bases were all present in equal amounts, and might therefore be arranged in a repeating sequence, but when more accurate analyses were made it turned out that the true situation is more complicated. The bases fall into pairs, A with T and G with C, and while the amount of A always equals that of T, and the amount of G equals that of C, the relative proportions of the two pairs vary from sample to sample. Each pair contains one large base, A or G, and one small one, T or C.

Evidence was also obtained that each sugar-phosphate chain in DNA is twisted like a runner bean round a pole, or a strand in a piece of thread, forming what is called a 'helix'. At first it was not known how many strands made up the thread, but eventually it was proved that there are two constituting a 'double helix'.

Now came the crucial step. By making scale models of the different parts of a DNA molecule and trying to fit them together – a thing chemists often do in the course of their researches – Dr. J. D. Watson and Dr. F. H. C. Crick, working in Cambridge, showed that there was just exactly room for an A – T or a G – C base-pair between the two strands of the double helix, but not for any of the other conceivable pairs, A – G, A – C, T – G or T – C. The pairing observed in practice thus found a natural explanation in terms of the sizes and shapes of the bases. This led Watson and Crick to the idea of a two-stranded structure, in which the strands are held together through their bases, an A on one strand forming a pair with a T on the other strand, and so on.

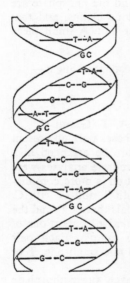

The idea of base-pairing carries with it a further implication of the utmost significance. It follows from it that each strand of DNA is complementary to the other. If the sequence of bases on one strand is known, then that on the other follows automatically. For instance ATGGCT on one strand implies TACCGA on the other – T opposite A, A opposite T, C opposite G, and so on. If therefore we take a single strand from the double helix and arrange for the separate sugar, phosphate and base units to build up on it to make a second strand again, then we shall have a copy of the

A molecule of DNA, showing the two twisted strands of the double helix, and the bases (marked A, C, G and T) between them.

original double helix. We can imagine doing this with either of the original single strands, and so obtain two double helices, each an exact copy of the original. In other words, in the presence of food in the form of sugar, phosphate and the four bases, DNA can in certain circumstances reproduce or replicate itself, and it can do this in full and precise detail, so that the progeny have the same sequence of bases as the parent. DNA possesses therefore one of the properties that we regard as characteristic of living things, the power to reproduce its own kind.

The Genetic Code

Seeing that a particular base-sequence is copied again and again by the mechanism just described, we naturally ask what significance we can attach to the actual sequences we find in living organisms. They might be mere random sequences that have arisen by chance, but this is unlikely in a biological context. It turns out in fact that the DNA molecule carries a message. Just as the groupings of dots and dashes in the Morse code convey information, so do the groupings of the four bases in the DNA molecule. The grouping ATG means one thing, the grouping GGC another, and the grouping CAG yet another. If the bases appearing along the length of the DNA molecule are divided up into successive groups of three, their message can be read like the message on a ticker tape.

The living cell possesses the machinery for reading the message. It converts it from its Morse code form into something like alphabetical form. The 'letters' of the alphabet are twenty substances called by the chemist 'amino acids', and known to be the constituents of the proteins of plant and animal bodies. Thus the base-grouping ATG is 'read' as the amino acid, methionine, GGC as glycine and CAG as glutamine. If the sequence ATGGGCCAG occurs in the DNA molecule, the cell will form a chain consisting of methionine linked to glycine linked to glutamine. Very long chains are built up in this way, and indeed that is how proteins are made. The scheme relating particular triads of bases to particular amino acids is the celebrated 'genetic code'.

We believe we have here the principal key to the construction of almost the entire plant or animal organism. The organism is made mainly of different kinds of protein, and each is a chain of amino acids arranged in a particular order. The properties of the protein derive from the order. Some kinds of amino acid chains form long bundles of fibres giving us our hairs, others form hard coverings, giving us our nails, others enable us to digest our food, and so on. The point is that the DNA molecule contains all the information or instructions needed to enable the cells of our bodies to piece these proteins together from the amino acids in digested food. For a number of proteins we know indeed the complete amino acid sequence, which is generally at least a hundred units in length.

There is nothing else remotely similar in the whole of chemistry. No other group of compounds carries anything like so much information as either DNA or the proteins. No molecule other than DNA has the power to pass on large amounts of information both to replicas of itself and to molecules of a different type, the proteins. No group but the proteins extracts such infinite variety of function from a single structural theme. Each separate facet of the picture is a wonder in itself, and the fact that the facets combine together in the way they do is an even greater wonder.

Synthesising Life

Now that the chemists have the necessary clues it is possible that they will be able to devise other types of compounds that can store and transmit large amounts of information, but it seems most unlikely that they will ever achieve in any other system the full combination of properties necessary for life. They may be able to create variants of the present-day DNA-protein system, and indeed such variants may have come into being during the early evolution of life, but the existence of any really distinct alternative (for instance based on the element silicon rather than carbon) seems improbable in the extreme.

One further feature of the DNA-protein system may be mentioned: DNA apparently cannot function on its own. It can neither replicate nor build proteins without the help of some of the very proteins it builds. It is not enough to provide it with the separate components needed for replication, the phosphate, sugar bases, or with the amino acids needed to form proteins. Certain pre-formed proteins must also be added to get the system started. Thus life as we know it depends on an interlocking scheme involving both DNA and proteins. This sets a pretty chicken-and-egg problem in evolutionary theory, to which we do not yet know the answer: which came first, DNA or proteins? or did they somehow arise together?

128

Life, Chemistry and Consciousness

The discovery of the role of DNA in life processes seems to have resolved one aspect of the long-standing controversy about vitalism. By vitalism is meant the idea that life cannot be fully explained in terms of physics and chemistry but involves some further 'life-force' or 'biotonic phenomenon' or what-have-you. Many have felt that vitalism leaves room in the world for freewill, morality and the things of the spirit, and have held on to it for that reason. The materialists have been equally determined to deny and sometimes to decry it. Our new knowledge seems to imply that so far as the material structure of our bodies is concerned, the information contained in the DNA molecule explains everything. Life is apparently based on chemistry – unique and extraordinary chemistry, but not different in basic principle from the rest of the subject.

There is of course an immense extrapolation in making claims of this kind. What we still have to learn is very much greater than what we know. Yet there is little doubt of the direction in which the available evidence points.

The idea that we might take a number of quite simple chemical substances, definitely non-living, and put them together in the laboratory to make life, no longer appears right outside the bounds of practicability. Indeed the synthesis of a virus from non-living material may be achieved quite soon. A virus lacks the full apparatus of a living cell, and may consist of no more than DNA and a single protein forming a coat. It cannot replicate except by entering a cell as a parasite and taking over the replicative machinery it finds there. Being so relatively simple it should be much easier to synthesise than any other form of life. The further step to a living cell is likely to be many orders of magnitude more difficult.

There is, however, no longer any difficulty about making a living cell as a thought-experiment. There is no longer any fundamental mystery about the working of the cell, to make us feel that something more is required than the right atoms in the right places, linked up in the right way. Nor is there any difficulty, in thought, about making all the cells and other constituents of a man's body and putting them together in the same positions as in his body. Even the brain is not to be excluded; it too consists of chemical substances obeying chemical and physical laws.

Mind and Consciousness

The question that springs to mind is then: if such a synthesis were carried out, would we then have a man? If we copied Mr X atom by atom, would we then have another Mr X?

Nobody can be sure of the answer. The Christian would doubt whether the synthetic Mr X would have a soul. The materialist, though he may pooh-pooh the soul, still has to face the problem of mind and consciousness. Would the synthetic Mr X have that inner life of thoughts, ideas, intuitions, feelings and emotions that I know from direct experience, and take it that you and the real Mr X know too? The materialist would presumably not expect to find any difference between the two Mr X's, but what then is this strange phenomenon of mind and consciousness?

Simply by studying matter – the structure of atoms, how their structure causes them to combine to form molecules, how simple molecules combine to give complicated molecules, how molecules come together to produce crystals, fibres, films and other structures, and finally how they produce living cells and multicellular organisms – we could hardly expect to arrive at the concept of consciousness. There seems to be an impossible jump in going from one world to the other. The difficulty is rather like that of describing the sensation of blueness to a completely colour-blind man. We may some day be able to tell him in precise terms what happens to the matter of our brains when we see the colour blue, but that would still not tell him what blue looks like to us. In the same way consciousness as an experience seems for ever beyond the reach of purely material description.

The existence of consciousness is a mystery enough in itself, but the mystery deepens when we ask how consciousness is related to the world of matter. The relationship is clearly of the most intimate and detailed kind. Much of the content of consciousness is derived from the material world through the senses. Light reaching our eyes produces pictures in our minds, pressure waves in the atmosphere produce sensations of sound, and so on. We can indeed go a step further and make the plausible assertion that through the eyes and the optic nerve light sets up a pattern of electric currents among the nerve-cells in the brain, and that this pattern is interpreted as a picture; and similarly with the other senses. The mystery lies at the last step in the chain in each case, at the point where we jump from a pattern of electric currents to their interpretation by the mind.

Is Freewill an Illusion?

There is also a relation between consciousness and the world of matter through our motor nerves and muscles. Here more may be involved than in the case of the senses. Through the senses our bodies record some sort of images of events in the external world, and our minds thereby become aware of them, but where muscular action is concerned the mind seems in addition to have some power of control. That at any rate is our naïve impression. We seem to have a measure of freewill, so that we can choose between, say, turning to the right or turning to the left. We also seem able to exert some degree of control over the contents of our consciousness; we can focus our attention here or there, or we can throw out one thought and accept another.

What is very difficult to see is how we can have any such freedom to choose and power to control without contravening the physical and chemical laws of matter. There seems indeed quite a widespread belief that the only way out is to regard freewill as an illusion; and if freewill goes, so does morality. On this view events in the material world feed our consciousness, so that our thoughts and feelings provide a sort of running commentary, but there is no feed-back in the opposite direction. The commentary is no more than a commentary; it adds nothing to the forces and laws that control matter. We could account for everything that happens to matter without bringing in consciousness at all. The technical term for this is 'epi-phenomenalism'; the mind and consciousness are said to be mere 'epi-phenomena'.

Is this the philosophy that physics and chemistry, rein-

E* 131

forced by the recent discoveries about DNA, force us to adopt? If so, we have indeed reached a devastating conclusion. To many philosophers, and to most of us in our everyday lives, the inner world of the mind has comparable status to the external world of matter. We treat them as equally significant aspects of a single reality. We explore both worlds, interpret events in both, develop theories about both, and by and large we appear to be able to make good sense of both. Is one of them really of utterly trivial significance?

At the present time it is not possible to point to scientific evidence that provides a conclusive refutation of epiphenomenalism, but it is possible to adduce strong reasons for doubting it. There is first the point that the epiphenomenalists carry on their everyday affairs as if they were making free choices all the time. It is indeed just about impossible to do anything else. Sometimes they even try with evangelistic fervour to convert others to their point of view, which seems absurd if the people they are trying to convert have no choice. Of course both their fervour and other people's responses may be chemically and physically determined, so that no actual contradiction is necessarily involved. The difficulty however is that if my philosophical views are the product of chemical and physical processes in my brain, what validity do they have? If they are 'given' by electric currents between the nerve-cells, why should they be either true or false? The conclusion seems to be that a philosophy that reduces my thought-life to an epiphenomenon is self-defeating.

We cannot escape from the dilemma by appealing to natural selection. We cannot argue that true thought-patterns will confer a greater benefit on the organism than false, so that an organism whose thoughts make sense will tend to survive at the expense of one whose thoughts are nonsense. This argument only holds water if our thoughts produce effects in the material world, since otherwise they cannot affect our survival. Yet such a feed-back from consciousness to the material world is the very thing the epiphenomenalist denies.

Another reason for caution in our attitude is that no

experiments have yet been made which might show in any direct way whether matter informed by mind behaves differently from unconscious matter. All the chemical experiments with DNA, for example, are carried out, so far as we can tell, in the absence of any form of consciousness in the material under investigation. It is like observing an orchestra performing without a conductor. Some orchestras produce most beautiful music in this way, and this might easily lead us to the false conclusion that the conductor is of no real significance, but merely follows with his baton the activities of the orchestra. The conclusion from studies of unconscious matter that consciousness is a mere epiphenomenon may be equally false.

The Nature of Matter

Perhaps however the strongest reason for caution is our ignorance of the nature of matter itself. We have come a long way from the little hard balls attracting and repelling one another that once seemed to provide such a solid foundation for our theories of the world. In probing ever more deeply into the nucleus of the atom, physicists have discovered not the ultimate simplicities of the universe, but strange and ill-understood complexities.

Even what we think is firm ground in our knowledge of matter is peculiar enough. For example according to the Heisenberg uncertainty principle any particle might be found anywhere in the universe, while according to the Pauli exclusion principle there is a sense in which every particle affects every other particle in the universe. Moreover we can never tell if the particle we observe at one moment of time is identical with the particle we observe at a later moment. It is not just a matter of the identification being difficult; the particles do not possess individual identities, and would obey different mathematical laws if they did.

By and large we ignore all these mysterious features when we study chemistry and molecular biology; we go back to the little hard balls, or to something rather like them. This is what Watson and Crick did when they discovered the secret of DNA. It is an approach that is highly successful in describing most, though not all, of the everyday forms of matter. To those immersed in it, this type of description may seem so successful that they are impatient of anyone who doubts its ability to give a full explanation of life. Yet in the present state of our knowledge it is a perfectly tenable view that some of the more recondite properties of matter come into play in a living organism, especially where mind is concerned.

To achieve a satisfactory synthesis between our experience of consciousness and our knowledge of matter remains a problem. Some suggestions as to how the two aspects of the world can be reconciled will be found in the next chapter. My aim has been to bring out the difficulties inherent in the plausible view that since the recent discoveries about DNA it is only a matter of time before life is fully explained by physics and chemistry.

Further reading

One of the best simple yet authoritative accounts of DNA and the genetic code is to be found in J. KENDREW: 'The Thread of Life' (Bell, 1966).

12

BRAIN AND PERSONALITY

Professor M. A. JEEVES, m.a., ph.d.

*Professor Jeeves, formerly of the University of
Adelaide, South Australia, now occupies the Chair of
Psychology at the University of St Andrews in
Scotland.*

In a letter to the first issue of a new international inter-
disciplinary journal devoted to developmental psycho-
biology, Dr H. Selye, well known for his pioneering researches into the effects of stress, wrote, 'Perhaps one of the
most important tasks of contemporary biology is to bridge
the gap between the psychic and the somatic manifestations
of life' (i.e. between mind and body). The subject matter
of this chapter lies at the heart of this relationship. The
relation of brain and personality raises issues concerned
with both psychosomatic and somatopsychic interrelations.

Today no widely read person can be unaware of the
intimate relationship between the workings of the human
brain and the way in which people behave. For some the
importance of this relationship is forcefully brought home
when a relative behaves abnormally because of a congenital
deformity of the brain, or a friend shows emotional or
mental changes after some insult to the brain through accident. Perhaps most common is the experience of watching
an ageing relative's memory change as degenerative processes in the brain slowly progress. It is encouraging that
intensive research directed at increasing our knowlege of
this relationship between brain and behaviour has already
brought considerable benefit to mankind in the treatment of
brain diseases and mental illness. Such research during the
past fifteen years has received fresh impetus through the
inter-disciplinary co-operation of neurologists, neuro-

surgeons, psychologists, psychiatrists, physiologists and bio-chemists. In the last ten years in particular, several inter-national meetings have been held which have brought to-gether leading workers in these fields to discuss not only specific problems concerning the functioning of the brain, but also some of the implications of this new knowledge for wider problems, ethical and moral. Some contributors at such meetings have drawn particular attention to the dangers inherent in such knowledge in that it opens the way for the manipulation of less well informed people by experts, or by ruthless politicians advised by such experts. Indeed, Aldous Huxley's *Brave New World* to some seems horrifyingly near to becoming a reality. Other participants have drawn attention to the fresh challenge which such knowledge brings to man's claim to exercise freedom of choice and action, both in his private affairs and in the affairs of groups and nations. Those concerned with this kind of problem have raised questions such as: if man's brain is as physically determinate as it appears to be, then what room remains for concepts such as choice and free will? Are these illusions left over from our ignorant past?

Before we can discuss these latter questions it will first be necessary to present a brief review, for the non-specialist, of some of the trends in contemporary research, which on the one hand increase our understanding of the intimate relationship between personality and brain struc-ture, and on the other hand, sharpen up some of the ethical problems which flow from new advances in the neuro-sciences. This done we shall discuss the broader issues which face man today and promise to become more urgent as neuroscientific knowledge steadily increases.

BRAIN AND PERSONALITY – AN INTIMATE RELATIONSHIP

An accident which occurred in September, 1848, to Phineas Gage, a foreman of a road construction gang working in America, demonstrated two things dramatically. First, that severe damage to the frontal lobes of the brain could have non-spectacular effects on mental processes such as memory, but second, that it could have spectacular effects on personality, producing marked changes in general attitudes towards the world, people and things. Gage was taking part in a routine blasting operation when unfortunately through failing to make the customary checks on his assistant's preparations, he inadvertently ignited a charge of powder which propelled an iron rod 4 feet long and $1\frac{1}{2}$ inches thick cleanly through his brain entering high in his left cheek and emerging from the top of his head. The amazing thing was that although Gage was stunned he was nevertheless able to walk to see a surgeon, recovered from the infection that developed in the wound and lived for another twelve years. Until that time it had been widely believed that the frontal lobes of the brain were the seat of the so-called higher intellectual processes, yet Gage displayed a remarkably small decrease in his mental capacities. It soon became clear, however, that his personality, rather than his intelligence, had been affected. Before the accident he had been considerate, efficient and well balanced, but afterwards he was irresponsible, fitful and irreverent, indulging frequently in gross profanity and manifesting little consideration for others. In addition he had become obstinate, capricious and vacillating. By demonstrating that the human brain in some respects is relatively invulnerable to extensive damage to a portion of it which had previously been considered to be of overriding importance, the case of Phineas Gage stimulated further medical research and led to more careful investigation of the effects of major brain damage.

The concept of personality is in rough terms intuitively meaningful to everyone. Whilst it is possible to find a wide range of precise definitions of personality in the writings of professional psychologists, it is fair to say that most psychologists would agree that the personality of an individual is that characteristic and relatively consistent pattern of behaviour which serves to distinguish him as an individual. By pattern of behaviour we mean, in non-technical terms, the sum total of the most important things that we can say about a person, the sort of things that make us like him or dislike him, or cause us to feel indifferent to his fate; personality thus includes what a man wants, what he will do to get it, and how he copes with his inability to get everything he needs and desires. It is also shown by the way a man is influenced by the circumstances in which he lives, and how he himself sets about influencing those same circumstances. For the purposes of analysis it is customary and useful to distinguish the determinants of personality according to two broad classes, the genetic and physiologically based on the one hand, and the social and culturally based on the other. Our task in this chapter is primarily to explore the former, concentrating on the relationship between the structure of the brain and the personality of the individual, although inevitably we shall have to say something about the interaction between these biological determinants and the environment in which the organism finds itself.

THE LINKS BETWEEN BRAIN AND PERSONALITY

For the benefit of the non-specialist we shall give some examples, familiar to neuroscientists, of the evidence from brain lesion studies, electrical stimulation studies and studies of brain chemistry, to illustrate the close linkage between the structure and functioning of the brain.

Evidence from Lesion Studies

Congenital or acquired abnormalities or lesions in the physical structure of the brain often play an important role in creating personality disturbances, not only because of the direct effect of change of brain structure on behaviour, but also because of problems of social adjustment which not infrequently flow from the problems created by the brain damage as such. That such behavioural and personality changes induced by lesions are dependent on the region predominantly affected may be illustrated by reference to the effects of damage to three parts of the brain, the frontal lobes, the temporal lobes, and the hypothalamus. The hemispheres of the brain are separated into parts by so-called sulci, which are depressions or intervals between folds or convolutions, known as gyri. Some sulci separate parts of the hemispheres called lobes. Each lobe supposedly has separate functions. Whilst to a certain extent this is true, it is nevertheless found that some such functional distinctions between lobes are much more arbitrary than was previously thought. The frontal lobe is in front of the central sulcus and the temporal lobe is below the lateral sulcus. The hypothalamus is a part of the so-called brain stem which lies below and between the cerebral hemispheres.

The kinds of symptoms associated with damage to the frontal lobes which were manifest in the case of Phineas Gage are still regarded as fairly typical of results of damage to that area of the brain. Many studies have supported the view that a person who previously might have been ambitious, well adjusted and highly motivated, will after frontal lobe damage lose his former drive, become insensitive to the feelings of others, disorganised, tactless and frequently manifest a general lack of responsiveness to ethical and moral considerations. Not infrequently there is also often a general feeling of euphoria reported by these persons. As is now widely known these changes brought about by damage to the frontal parts of the brain can be put to positive use in restoring the balance where a person has become chronically depressed and over-anxious. For a time the surgical procedures of either pre-frontal lobotomy or leucotomy were used fairly widely with psychiatric patients with whom all other procedures seemed to have failed. Patients selected for this procedure today usually show chronic agitation and severe distress, persistent depression, emotional aggression and excited and impulsive behaviour. The operation has been shown to relieve phobias, obsessions, hallucinations and delusions which are not of long standing duration.

In 1937 Kluver and Bucy described a behavioural syndrome in Rhesus monkeys which followed bilateral surgical lesions of the temporal lobes. This syndrome was characterised by alterations in the emotional behaviour of the animals. Further developments of this work indicated how wild irascible animals may become tame and docile and at the same time may display increased but poorly differentiated sexual activity. It is now evident that the full story about temporal lobe functioning is going to be very much more complex than was earlier thought. For example, the amygdala, embedded deep within the temporal lobes, have been found to be closely associated with expressions of fear and rage. In animals, damage to selected parts of this region of the brain has led to fearlessness, but even this change is complicated in that it is related to social factors, such as the position that a monkey holds in the dominance hierarchy of its group before surgical intervention. In one study specific decreases in dominance behaviour were reported to occur only in monkeys which had previously held their dominance rank by persistent challenge, indicating an interaction between nervous system function and social behaviour. Evidence concerning the effect of lesions in this area of the brain is further complicated by the finding that the placidity resulting from bilateral amygdalectomy can be converted into vicious rage by a further lesion in the nearby ventromedial nucleus of the hypothalamus (Shreiner and Kling, 1953). The point is that these experiments, with many others, reveal the complexity of brain-behaviour interactions in animals and serve as a warning that many factors as yet not understood at all may have to be considered in attempted surgical modifications of personality through manipulation of the brain in humans. Fully aware of the grave responsibility they carry, some neurosurgeons in recent years have attempted to bring relief from intractable behaviour disorders in children by means of lesions in the amygdala. Needless to say such operations are undertaken only as a last resort, but successes so far achieved justify cautious optimism for similar developments in the future.

Much of the early work on brain-behaviour relationships other than that on the cortex was concerned with the hypothalamus and it is now clear that this structure is primarily concerned with the integration of emotional behaviour, regulating as it does the autonomic nervous system, endocrine balance and temperature adjustments. Since the early experiments of Masserman in 1943 views have changed considerably, but it still remains clear that one fundamental role which the hypothalamus plays is in the control of sexual behaviour. In animals, anterior hypothalamic lesions appeared to eliminate sexual behaviour completely, whilst stimulation of the same area electrically produced persistent ejaculation or oestrous behaviour.

Evidence from Electrical Stimulation Studies

The advances in the development of neurosurgical procedures now make it possible to allow human subjects to report experiences resulting from electrical stimulation of various cortical areas. Such techniques are not only of importance clinically but also reveal more of brain-personality linkages. Pioneering studies in this area are associated with the name of Wilder Penfield and his work on the temporal lobes. More recently self-stimulation experiments have added evidence of a physiological influence of special areas of brain on behaviour. For example, the original observations of Olds and Milner (1954) indicated that when certain areas in the brains of rats were stimulated electrically, such stimulation acted as a positive reinforcement to behaviour. Thus an animal would continue to press a lever which gave rise to electrical stimulation through electrodes implanted in its brain, in a way similar to the bar pressing behaviour elicited by food or other positive rewards. Subsequent research with humans and animals has revealed reinforcing properties of considerable strength in the brain stem and hypothalamus in particular. Human subjects in such experiments are usually patients with epilepsy, mental illness or brain tumours. Areas of positive reinforcement in subcortical regions such as the septal region and amygdala also elicit a variety of subjective impressions. Descriptions of the effects of such stimulation vary from feelings of general well being, to specific pleasurable sensations (Lilly, 1960). Stimulation of other areas often in close juxtaposition to positive reinforcement areas produced disagreeable or painful sensations, whereas many areas including most of the neo-cortex appear neutral in this respect.

Evidence from Studies of Brain Chemistry

The deficiency or excess of various chemicals naturally occurring in the body may enable us to relate such chemistry of the brain to personality changes (Nurnberger *et al.*, 1963). For example the vitamins thiamine and niacin are

141

particularly important in this respect. Deficiency of thiamine causes disturbances in sleep, loss of appetite, lethargy and fatiguability. Niacin deficiency causes similar symptoms and in addition impairment in memory, orientation and intellectual functioning generally. The influence of these chemicals on the brain is obvious, and associated personality changes hinge on these defects.

As is well known a variety of hormone deficiencies can also produce changes in personality. Evidence is accumulating that various neuro-hormones, that is hormones which seem to play a special role in the proper functioning of the central nervous system, may participate in the etiology, pathogenesis or manifestation of some mental disorders. To take one example, serotonin is a neuro-hormone present in the central nervous system, in particular in the mid-brain and hypothalamus (Bogdanski and Udenfriend, 1956). Serotonin does not itself readily cross the so-called blood-brain barrier which prevents substances in the blood from entering the brain, but an amino-acid from which it can readily be formed, can enter the brain and there be converted by a process of decarboxylation into serotonin. The amino-acid in question, known as 5-hydroxytryptophan, when administered intravenously causes marked excitement and autonomic disturbances in dogs and other experimental animals (Udenfriend *et al.*, 1957). This is important when considering results from investigations of certain antidepressant drugs which inhibit the action of another substance, monamine oxidase, which is also present in the body and in turn destroys serotonin by turning it into 5-hydroxyindole acetic acid, suggesting that such drugs may acquire their antidepressant properties by increasing brain serotonin (Bogdanski *et al.*, 1958). This implies that serotonin may have a possible role in minimising depression. We cannot pursue the details here, but the point remains that the implied linkage between brain and personality, whilst not direct, is too evident to be ignored. The very large volume of psychopharmacological work published in recent years is certainly sufficient to enable us to conclude that a definite linkage exists between brain and personality at the biochemical level.

ENVIRONMENTAL CONDITIONS, BRAIN FUNCTIONING
AND PERSONALITY

The work of H. Selye has already become widely known and may be treated as a good example of relevant work in this area. One general conclusion from his work is that anxiety can have widespread effects on the physiology of the organism, and that it may be possible to understand neurosis as partly a matter of altered physiological state. If this turns out to be true it certainly represented an important brain-personality link up. Experiments have shown that both physical and psychological stress activate the pituitary gland, in part through the neuro-secretory activity of the hypothalamus referred to earlier. The pituitary in turn releases hormones which activate other endocrine glands of the body, particularly the adrenal cortex. Once stressed, this system may become sensitive to additional stresses, and two kinds of disorder may occur, first an early one due to over-secretion of the adrenal gland and possibly contributing to such psychosomatic symptoms as hypertension; and a second one due to adrenal exhaustion and perhaps contributing to symptoms of rheumatism and arthritis, also believed to be partly psychosomatic in origin. Whilst many of these notions are still speculative, their relevance to this discussion is that they draw attention to a physiological principle which seems to be at work and which indicates ways in which prolonged emotional stress may affect the physiology of the organism and sensitise it to further emotional disturbances. For instance in the study of gastric ulcers evidence is accumulating that environmental factors are responsible for prolonged chemical changes in gastric fluids (Brady *et al.*, 1958). Whilst precise relationships between cause and effect are not known, nevertheless central structures important to the autonomic nervous system are probably involved such as the hypothalamus and the pituitary gland.

Another area of research which has received a good deal of publicity in recent years can be exemplified by the work of Thompson and Melzack (1956) who found that puppies socially isolated from litter mates and other animals from seven to ten months after birth retained quite immature forms of behaviour for fairly long periods thereafter. In a related study Seitz (1959) has observed effects of social isolation on learning in kittens, when isolation was introduced in the second to sixth week of life. In this instance however the isolated animals were in general more vigilant, alert and aggressive than non-isolated controls. Mason (1960) found somewhat similar effects on social behaviour in the Rhesus monkey. Rosenzweig, Krech and Bennett (1958, 1962, 1964) in a series of papers have also explored the effects of early environment upon later behaviour and more specifically upon brain structure. On reaching maturity those animals that were reared from birth in an enriched environment differed markedly from those that were reared in an impoverished environment not only in behaviour but also in brain weight and brain biochemistry.

The examples cited in the sections above have been chosen, not because they are necessarily the most important, but because they are ones which may already be familiar to the widely read layman and which are sufficient to indicate the close relationship between the physical state of the brain and the behaviour and personality of the organism possessing that brain. The studies on the effects of environment on brain and behaviour are perhaps particularly important, since they can be taken to imply that the attitudes that a man adopts towards other people and towards circumstances may result in an increase or reduction in stress and anxiety, which in turn may produce changes in the brain either of a temporary or permanent nature. It is of course this very close relationship between the structure of the brain and the personality and behaviour of the person, that have led some to argue that if the brain is indeed a physically determinate system, then to speak, as we still do, of freedom of choice, is quite misleading, since such freedom is merely illusory. Others have looked at the same evidence and said that it underlines what many have said for a long time, namely, that the attitudes which we adopt are of prime importance since they are reflected in the physical state of the body, not only in temporary variations but also in more permanent changes, and, they argue, this gives added importance to what many religious people maintain about the importance of appropriate attitudes towards people and circumstances. It is to these more philosophical but nonetheless important questions, that we must now turn briefly.

The steadily increasing knowledge of the physical functioning of the brain has sharpened up the issues that arise when the common belief in man's individual freedom is re-examined in the light of such knowledge. It has not only been the philosophers and the religious men who have raised these questions, but many of the leading neuroscientists themselves have been concerned to offer solutions to the problems which arise when due weight is given to the evidence which points more and more clearly towards a view which regards the brain as essentially a deterministic physical mechanism. Not many years ago in a symposium of British scientists there seemed to be a wide measure of agreement that the neural activity of the brain somehow interacts with the private world of the mind (see *The Physical Basis of Mind* edited by P. Laslett).

As a good example of this sort of view, which has been carefully developed, we may consider the suggestion made by Eccles, a Nobel prizeman and distinguished neurophysiologist, that 'the mind-brain liaison occurs in the cortex'. According to this view, first presented in 1951, the will of man can influence neural circuits without violating physical laws because the energy involved in such influence is within the limits of what is known as the Heisenberg Uncertainty principle. Eccles suggests that there might be an influence of the mind on individual quantum events in the brain, whose effects can then be amplified through other parts of the cortex, or more probably there could be a coordinated effect on many such events simultaneously. In either case the picture is of neural activity being changed by non-physical factors. It is of interest that in some of Eccles' more recent writings, e.g. in the proceedings of a symposium on *Brain and Conscious Experience* held in

1965, he appears to be changing his views somewhat. It has been pointed out that Eccles' 1951 view does not give due weight to the fact that the degree of physical indeterminacy allowed by Heisenberg's principle becomes more and more negligible the bigger the objects that are being studied. Indeed it is only with the smallest objects of all, electrons for example, that this indeterminacy is really serious and although a nerve cell may be a tiny object by everyday standards it is roughly a million million million times heavier than an electron, so that the chances of its suffering appreciably from Heisenberg indeterminacy are small indeed. It has also been pointed out that the random variations in the brain due to the kind of fluctuations that Heisenberg has discussed may turn out to be quite small compared with other sorts of random variations, due for example to changes in the temperature of the brain tissue, random fluctuations in the blood supply and other kinds of disturbances reaching the brain from the outside world. But the most serious objection to this view is one which has been emphasised by MacKay (1967), who pointed out that 'if an element of randomness came into the chain of control of my action, this would tend towards *excusing* me from responsibility for it rather than crediting me with responsibility for it'. To put it more bluntly, such a view would provide excellent grounds for acting irresponsibly because one could then attribute actions considered ethically or morally unacceptable to one or more neurones firing randomly without oneself being in agreement with such firing. Most recently MacKay in a number of places, but in greatest detail in his 1967 Eddington Memorial Lecture, has expounded an approach to this problem, which whilst giving full weight to the evidence supporting the view that the brain should be regarded as essentially a physically determinate system, at the same time spells out the implications of this for freedom of choice and action. MacKay concludes that if the brain is physically determinate this does not *ipso facto* rule out the possibility of freedom of action. MacKay's argument is not easy to follow and readers are advised to refer to his detailed statement of it in the Eddington Lecture.

However in the following paragraph the essential points of his argument will be set out in summary form.

MacKay begins by pointing out the need to distinguish carefully between two possible meanings of the word 'free'. If by free we mean unpredictable by anyone, then on the hypothesis we are considering there is no such thing as freedom because a super-scientist who has full knowledge of the present physical state of your brain plus environment, and of the equations upon which its future activity is based, can predict its future state. MacKay argues, however, that the kind of freedom we need for the idea of responsibility to have meaning and relevance is somewhat different. Thus he writes, 'to call an action free is therefore to deny the existence of any determinate specification that is binding on (valid and definitive for) everyone, including the *agent,* before he makes up his mind. It is this kind of freedom that I suggest underlies human responsibility'. On this view we need to be able to say that if I am to be responsible for a choice, then no inescapable determinative prediction must exist which is equally binding on me whether I know it or not, whether I believe it or not, and whether I like it or not.

In developing his argument MacKay asks us to imagine a super-scientist who studies the state of my brain, and who then knowing the present conditions plus the equations that summarise the operating characteristics of my brain, makes a prediction concerning a decision which I am about to make in a given situation. Of course by definition if he keeps quiet about his prediction, and if he is in fact a super-scientist, he will be able to sit back and see his prediction fulfilled. An experiment of this kind, however, will prove nothing one way or the other about my ability to choose or not my freedom; it will simply prove that the super-scientist really was super! In what sense, may we ask, is his prediction a true prediction? To put the question in another way, what does he suggest that I would have been correct to believe at the time when he made his prediction? If his prediction had the same inevitability as the forecast of an eclipse, for example, then it should be correct whether I see it or not, whether I believe it or not, and whether I like it or not. Predictions about behaviour, on the other hand, turn out to be fundamentally different for the following reasons. According to the mechanistic determinist's own assumptions, derived from the kind of evidence reviewed earlier in this chapter, whatever I believe is rigorously reflected in the state of my brain. It follows then that no complete description of the state of my brain can exist which would be equally correct whether or not I believed it, since my believing it would (on the same assumptions) be reflected in a change in that state. The point is that whatever prediction the super-scientist may write on paper, if it is to be valid for him it cannot be equally valid for me – I would in fact be mistaken to believe it, since my believing it would change the state of my brain in such a way that it no longer corresponded to the description of the brain state upon which the prediction was based. In fact, whatever else you may say about the prediction on the paper, for me it has no binding force; it has no inevitable claim on my assent, whether I know it or not, whether I believe it or not, and whether I like it or not. As MacKay has put it, 'the key point is that if what a man believes affects correspondingly the state of his organising system, no complete up-to-date account of that organising system could be believed by him without being *ipso facto* rendered out of date'. It is important to remember that this argument is not at all based upon a question of our ignorance of brain processes. It is an inevitable corollary of any theory, however deterministic, that assumes that our thinking is rigorously reflected in the workings of our brain, and as MacKay continues, 'Even if brain functions were as mechanical as clockwork (which they are not), our choices would have this "built-in indeterminacy" which allows no advance prediction of them to be binding upon us.'

To sum up, the kind of evidence indicating a close relationship between the brain and personality which was presented in the early part of this chapter, even though it may well point to a mechanistic explanation of human brain activity, does not thereby eliminate our freedom. Those who urge mechanistic behaviourism so as to abolish moral and spiritual categories seem to be pursuing an illusion.

148

WIDER ISSUES

As the accelerating pace of research in the neurosciences and in medicine adds to our understanding of the structure and function of the brain, it also holds out high hopes that with further advances some of the suffering at present experienced by so much of mankind because of brain dysfunction will slowly give way to therapeutic measures which will relieve this suffering. The research worker who is a Christian will see this as added motivation for him to fulfil with renewed vigour his commission 'to subdue the created order' so that mankind may benefit from that which God has give us in creation. Men of many other religions, and humanists also, will from different presuppositions, but all motivated by the same concern for the well-being of mankind, be able to share in this endeavour. Thus, for example, our knowledge of the detrimental effects of things like impoverished environment, stress and anxiety, should increase the efforts of those concerned to bring about more widespread acceptance of positive attitudes. Such attitudes will in turn relieve suffering and avoid permanent injury to the brain which would otherwise be reflected in personalities which are cramped and stunted or deviant in various ways. Perhaps the most obvious and glaring example of an issue on which immediate action could be taken is that of malnutrition. There is now abundant evidence that some forms of malnutrition, especially in small children, result in changes to the structure and biochemistry of the brain which, if they occur at a critical period, may well be irreversible. The net result is the prospect of millions growing up with mental capacities and personality resources less than they could have been, had the right kind of food been made available at the right time.

As regards problems which arise concerning the manipulation of behaviour, some scientists, notably B. F. Skinner, have pointed out that already the knowledge that we have of the relation between brain and behaviour is sufficient to present a danger, in that the rapid development of new techniques in the control of behaviour may quickly outstrip the counter controls, which in most countries at the moment prevent exploitation by the use of force and deception. Despite objections there is no doubt that science will increasingly facilitate the control of human behaviour and it must be used wisely if we are to avoid disaster. In spite of the massive increase in research in psycho-pharmacology, examples of which were cited earlier, it seems at present that there is little likelihood of the deliberate use of any of the known psychoactive drugs for the control of behaviour of normal people. It is true that there have been many suggestions that drugs have been employed extensively in brain washing procedures in communist controlled countries. However, it is fair to say that from the reliable evidence available at the present time this does not seem to be the case. What is the case, according to reliable reports, is that where coercion of persons for the purpose of extracting confession is required, the methods that have been used are police state practices which have been used in various forms since the time of Napoleon. As regards the psychosurgical procedures mentioned earlier, some of which may bring distinct benefit to certain individuals, it is difficult to see how any practical application of them in the future could enable men deliberately to control each other's behaviour in any socially significant way on a large scale. One other field of neuroscientific research which we have not had time to develop in any detail is the study of learning and memory and their relationship to the structure of the brain. It may well be that in the not too distant future some of these studies will have practical applications in education and by the same token will be available for exploitation of the public by propagandists.

Finally, a note of warning needs perhaps to be sounded. Sufficient has been said in this chapter to indicate ways in which the personality of man is dependent upon the physical structure of the brain including its biochemistry, to suggest how such knowledge more fully developed could be abused and become an extremely powerful weapon in the hands of any minority group who wished to use it, not for the betterment of mankind, but rather to subjugate the mass of mankind to fulfil the will and purposes of a minority. This should surely underline the necessity for Christians, humanists, men of other religions and all men of goodwill, to ensure that high principles and clearly held ethical standards predominate in the affairs of men at all levels, including the application of increasing knowledge in the neurosciences.

REFERENCES

D. F. BOGDANSKI AND S. UDENFRIEND: 'Serotonin and monamine oxidase in brain'. *J. Pharmacol. & Exper. Therap.*, 1956, 116, 7.

D. F. BOGDANSKI, H. WEISSBACH AND S. UDENFRIEND: 'Biochemical findings relating to the action of serotonin'. *Ann. New York Acad. Sci.*, 1957, 66, 602.

J. V. BRADY, R. W. PORTER, D. G. CONRAD AND J. W. MASON: 'Avoidance behaviour and the development of gastroduodenal ulcers'. *J. exp. Anal. Behav.*, 1958, 1, 69-73.

J. C. ECCLES: 'Brain and Conscious Experience' (Springer-Verlag, New York, 1966).

H. KLUVER AND P. C. BUCY: 'Preliminary analysis of functions of the temporal lobes in monkeys'. *Archives of neurology and psychiatry*, 43, 979-1000

P. LASLETT (Ed.): 'The Physical Basis of Mind' (Blackwell, Oxford, 1952).

J. LILLY: 'The psychophysiological basis for two kinds of instincts'. *J. Amer. Psychoanal. Ass.*, 1960, 8, 659.

D. M. MACKAY: 'Freedom of Action in a Mechanistic Universe' (Cambridge University Press, 1967).

W. A. MASON: 'The effect of social restriction on the behaviour of rhesus monkeys: I, Free social behaviour'. *J. comp. Physiol. Psychol.*, 1960, 53, 582-589.

J. I. NURNBERGER, C. B. FERSTER AND J. P. BRADY: 'An introduction to the science of human behaviour' (Appleton-Century-Crofts, New York, 1963).

J. OLDS AND P. MILNER: 'First reports of areas of positive reinforcement in rat brain'. *J. comp. Physiol. Psychol.*, 1954, 47, 419.

M. R. ROSENZWEIG, E. L. BENNETT AND D. KRECH: Cerebral effects of environmental complexity and training among adult rats' *J. Comp. Physiol. Psychol.*, 1964, 57, 438-439.

M. R. ROSENZWEIG, D. KRECH AND E. L. BENNETT: 'Brain chemistry and adaptive behaviour'. In: H. F. HARLOW AND C. N. WOOLSEY (Eds.): 'Biological and Biochemical Bases of Behaviour' (University of Wisconsin Press, Madison, 1958).

M. R. ROSENZWEIG, D. KRECH AND E. L. BENNETT: 'Effects of environmental complexity and training on brain chemistry and anatomy'. *J. Comp. Physiol. Psychol.*, 1962, 55, 429-437.

L. SCHREINER AND A. KLING: 'Behavioural changes following rhinencephalic injury in cat'. *J. Neurophysiol.*, 1953, 16, 643

P. F. D. SEITZ: 'Infantile experience and adult behaviour in animal subjects: II, Age of separation from the mother and adult behaviour in the cat'. *Psychosom. Med.*, 1959, 21, 353-378.

W. R. THOMPSON AND R. MELZACK: 'Early environment' *Sci. Amer.*, 1956, 194, 38-42.

S. UDENFRIEND, H. WEISSBACH AND D. F. BOGDANSKI: 'Pharmacological studies with the serotonin precursor, 5-hydroxytryptophan'. *J Pharmacol. & Exper. Therap.*, 1958, 122, 182.

13

DISEASE AND HUMAN BEHAVIOUR

DONALD ROBERTSON,
M.B., CH.B., F.R.C.S., D.T.M. & H.

*Dr Robertson is Senior Lecturer in the Department
of Anatomy at the University Medical School in
Edinburgh, and has practised in Britain, Iraq and India.*

I want to start by presenting some very simple considerations, which anyone can easily grasp, and to illustrate them by stories and case-histories that are equally easy to follow. But nobody should be misled by the simplicity of what I have to say into overlooking the power and depth of the ideas in question. Some of them may seem familiar, even hackneyed, yet their value had been proved time and again in practice. Moreover they stand opposed at many points to views that are widely diffused in the medical profession today. Indeed they compel a good deal of rethinking, particularly in the realm of psychology and psychiatry, and in the later part of this chapter I shall indicate the kind of lines on which this rethinking may take place.

Conflict, Cause of Sickness

Somewhere in the mind of every doctor there is always the question: why do only some people become ill?

When I was responsible for twelve hundred families I constantly had to ask that question. Ninety per cent of the sickness came from a small group of families, whose children had one illness after another. What was the common factor, the likely causative factor? In every case save one there was in the family an over-anxious parent, and sometimes there were two. But there seemed to be one outstanding exception which required investigation.

I called on that family. We discussed the health of the

children; how colds and sore throats were seldom absent from one or other of the three youngsters. We spoke of their intestinal upsets and of how they were quick to become ill but slower than average to recover. We asked the question, 'Why?' There was no suggestion of neglect. They were well fed, warmly clothed and adequately cared for. I spoke of other families who had more than their share of illness, and said, 'I associate this with over-anxious parents, but you and your wife seem confident and at peace. Can you suggest anything?' He smiled across at his wife. 'Yes!' he said. 'My wife is a better actress than you realise. She is full of worry about the children's health. What do you suggest?'

The wife agreed. Then after some talk she saw that fear is really a hidden demand. She not only desired but demanded constant health for her children. She then accepted that God cared for them, but that illness might come, and she decided to accept whatever the future might bring as His will. This act of trust brought her great release and the children's health improved markedly.

Such families logically compelled my interest in the diseases we call psychosomatic. Born in the mind of man they are related to man's character and the mental climate of families. As we become more successful, with antibiotics, at conquering disease due to serious infection, they account for an increasing proportion of our cases. Let us look closely at such illness.

People use illness to attain a variety of conscious ends. 1) Many people when in a difficult situation use sickness to escape from it. I recall two men who were in charge of a hospital, and whose personalities clashed. One had six months of amoebic dysentery and escaped from the situation. Frequently in his mind had come the thought, 'If because of this infection I have to go I will not be blamed.'

During the Second World War many cases of amoebiasis arose in one tropical area and a number of trained officers were sent home. Then an order was published that all further cases would be treated locally until cured. The number of cases diminished dramatically. In my present teaching job it is noticeable that in the days before the examinations poor students frequently go off sick with upper respiratory or intestinal upsets; good students very seldom.

2) Another use of illness is to attract sympathy. This is very clear in many cases of asthma, intestinal upsets, and skin diseases. This is known to and observed by all and requires less discussion.

3) Recurrent attacks of symptoms are used to control others, especially in families. Recently a friend of mine told me his symptoms and then said, comfortably, 'My daughter is on holiday. She will come home and nurse me.' How often we have seen neuritis, colitis and so-called cardiac pain used to maintain control of a wife, a husband or a child.

4) Some make a protest by being ill. How many attacks of headache or migraine spring from this? A student said to me, 'I've had migraine over the weekend.' I asked, 'Why?' He said, 'I've got behind with my work. I always get it then. Now I'm working hard I won't have it again.' Illness which comes when we do not get our own way may well be a form of protest.

Effects of Hate, Fear and Greed

It is customary in this day and age to give neutral, inoffensive labels, and 'psychosomatic' is such a label. It excuses everything but cures nothing. There is no movement in it towards health. Let us instead speak of illness due to fear, hate and greed, because to do so demands action, change, cure.

Fear can be a factor in many diseases but outstandingly in asthma, peptic ulcers, and lesser intestinal disorders. In the days before steroids were available I had a patient with asthma. The attacks were very frequent, fairly severe and had occurred over a period of thirty-one years. I had failed to find a drug to bring cure. One morning I was thinking about her and I thought, 'Why not tackle her fears?' I asked her if she had any special fear in her life and she said, 'Yes!' 'But,' she added, 'I've had the fear for thirty-one years and I'll tell nobody about it.' Since her asthma had lasted a similar period this was suggestive, and I put it to her that she should consider the matter.

I saw her a week later, when she told me she could do

nothing. Her fear was that her husband would find out about an incident that had taken place thirty-one years previously. I suggested she should tell him and ask forgiveness, adding that he might have some unhappy secrets too which would be better discussed. 'Oh no!' she said. 'He would be angry and leave me.' On this note I had to leave.

Next week she was not only free from asthma but looked a free, happy person. She said, looking a little foolish, 'I've spoken to my husband. Do you know what he said? He said "I knew about that at the time but thought you didn't want to discuss it."' Not only was her asthma cured, but their life together became freer and richer.

There was a different outcome in the case of a middle-aged man with a duodenal ulcer. His surgeon explained that by operation he could be cured. 'But,' he said, 'you don't need operation. Your trouble is fear and worry. Why not go to your minister, talk over your fears and make a new start? I'll give you twenty-four hours to think it over.' Next day the patient said, 'Doctor, I'll hae ma stomach oot!' Did he, one wonders, think that his clerical friend would be quite unable to help, or was he afraid that he would be only too efficient? The surgeon performed the gastrectomy.

When we think of hate we naturally turn to rheumatoid arthritis. Resentment and jealousy are known to be major elements in this disease. A case known to the writer is now after many years slowly burning itself out. He was and is a deeply bitter man. When asked about it he agreed that his hands flared up when his life went sour. But he justified it. 'Do you wonder at it,' he asked, 'when my daughter died of starvation when I was unemployed in the thirties?' It is no use blaming such a patient; but had he stopped fighting a bitter class war in his heart and will, improvement would have swiftly come – possibly cure. He could still have fought to right the wrongs of the world, but without rancour.

Resentment can also cause other types of illness. A medical officer in my hospital was given full investigation for gastric pain. Nothing was found. In conversation he said, 'I know I have pain because I'm mad at the authorities who promised me leave and have not given it.' The pain then ceased and six weeks later he got his leave.

Greed is a more obvious cause of sickness. Greed for food leads to overweight; greed for sex to venereal disease and to conflict due to obsessions; greed for success to strain and cardio-vascular disease; greed for alcohol and tobacco to well-known *sequelae*. What is less well-known is that man may become free from greed, of all kinds, and move out of obsession into freedom. This is not moving into a stern ascetic life, narrow and limited. It is moving from a self-centred compulsive existence out to a purposeful redirection of energy, satisfying and socially effective. It is more blessed to give than to receive.

The Key to Cure

The question of course arises: how does a busy doctor, or anyone else, find time to deal with such cases? It takes much less time than we sometimes think, and we can make an experimental approach.

When I first became aware of the importance of psycho-somatic disease a friend suggested I would be more effective if I was consciously in touch with God's will. I did not believe this to be possible, but he said, 'You say you are scientist. Why not make the experiment?' The experiment was to take the first part of the day to listen, seeking illumination in the first place about my own motives. Some say to listen to the living God. Some say you can listen and as the days pass you will know from where the thoughts come.

The experiment was fruitful. Honesty began to reveal the springs of conduct in me and I saw how I had myself on occasion used illness to evade difficulties; how gastric pain came while I hesitated over a major decision. As honesty showed up my own motives so came insight into those of my patients. It also began to be clear how purity of life and thought released energy, bound in obsessive habits, for socially creative activity.

About this time an elderly man came asking for help. He was worried, his face was lined, he was guilt-ridden. There was in his nature a streak of the sexual deviant from which he sought release. First he became honest, and for the first time agreed that he *liked* his obsessive day-dream.

Then he became willing to give it up. Thirdly he, in quiet listening, sought God's will. He then said, 'I must give this to God not only for now but for the rest of my life.' On his knees he did just that. To my astonishment when he rose up he looked ten years younger. The lined face had in a moment smoothed out. His wife could hardly believe her eyes as he told her. From then on he became a creative force in his business community and passed on to many the secret he had found. This and similar experiences taught me that God's standards of honesty and purity are absolute, and that each can know for himself what that involves.

The experiment of listening naturally leads to an expansion of mind and thought. It is not a passive experience: our best thinking and most active questioning are enhanced by a wisdom greater than our own. We find insight and the will to action. From it may come the question which can expose the conflict behind the disease.

This analysis implies that what a man thinks and feels affects his susceptibility to infection. It also shows that he may by decisions of the will choose to step from obsession and introspection to freedom, from mental habits that make illness likely to those that bring health. The process is a conscious one, and the doctor can help the patient to take the right road. Moreover in so far as it is a matter of dealing with fear, hate and greed, and of an approach to God, the art should not be limited to the medical profession; the teacher, the clergyman, everyone involved in industrial relations, and indeed every member of any family can exercise it.

Freudianism in the Melting Pot

We have here a fundamental challenge to fifty years of thought stemming originally mostly from Freud, Jung and Adler, and now familiar not only as a means of therapy, but often as a way of life and as a considerable vested interest as well. Must all this go into the melting pot? Many think it must. Eysenck has claimed after examining the statistics that there is no evidence that on balance the established methods are beneficial to the patient. Cattell[1] suggests that history will look back to the age of Freud, Jung and Adler and say it 'amounted scientifically almost to a disaster in that the impressive facade of pseudo-knowledge took away the incentive to make those more modest experiments on which the advance of science depends'. Briefly then let us review the past fifty years and see if today a more hopeful future beckons.

How many of us can remember the optimism of the twenties? They were days of technical advance. The first hormone had been synthesized; the road to effective drugs was being opened up; the way to penicillin, though we were blind to it, had been laid down. But it was in psychology and education that optimism was most bold and facile. Many of us accepted Freud and his disciples as the liberators of our day. Some of us, alas, wanted this new philosophy because it would allow us to live as we wished.

To quote Aldous Huxley,[2] 'The liberation we desired was simultaneously liberation from a certain political and economic system and liberation from a certain system of morality. We objected to the morality because it interfered with our sexual freedom; we objected to the political and economic system because it was unjust.' Arguing our consciences to death we turned to Almighty Man. In the new psychology we sought a panacea.

Doctors, novelists, playwrights and even some clergy welcomed the new teaching. Educators rethought their philosophy. Ideologists wove the new psychology into their dialectic.

It entered the home with devastating effect. Many of the conflicts arising later in adult life were blamed on the parents, and parents consequently lost confidence and withdrew from their rightful place of authority. The bill for this is now being paid, a bill of very considerable magnitude.

Whole generations have been used as guinea pigs, as is now by implication admitted. Speaking of the attempts to apply the new philosophy to childhood Anna Freud says,[3] 'When we look back over their history now, after a period of more than forty years, we see them as a long series of trials and errors.' She then lists a series of emphases successively stressed by workers in this field. At one time 'full sexual enlightenment at an early age was advocated'.

Later 'when the new instinct theory gave aggression the status of a basic drive, tolerance was extended also to the child's early and violent hostilities.' When anxiety was deemed more important, 'Every effort was made to lessen the children's fear of parental authority.' Then came a time when guilt was emphasised and 'this was followed by the ban on all educational measures likely to produce a severe super-ego.'

Summing up with considerable frankness she makes the following statement, 'Some pieces of advice given to parents over the years were consistent with each other, others were contradictory and mutually exclusive. In short, in spite of many partial advances, psycho-analytic education did not succeed in becoming the preventive measure it set out to be.'

But this varying advice did have other results. It confused many parents, making them afraid to trust their own judgements. It may have been a major factor in the abdication from responsibility so disastrous today. It has led to a society with little will to tackle its own problems, and small sense of right and wrong.

Sigmund Freud put forward a technique claimed to be therapeutic which glorified pleasure and advocated permissiveness. In a well-known quotation he said, 'We have found it impossible to give our support to conventional morality which demands more sacrifices than it is worth.'

The new psychologists also propagated a new kind of irresponsibility. The philosophy of J. M. Barrie's *Dear Brutus,* as expressed in the quotation, 'The fault, dear Brutus, is not in our stars, but in ourselves that we are underlings,' is not for them. Man, for them, is what he is because of what happened to him in his early childhood. Later in life, they say, this can be modified a little, but transformation of character is not possible. The aim of therapy is apparently to enable the patient to understand, accept and live with his problems. Society, we are told, should accept this and condone.

If this is a correct and true philosophy of life, and a wise method of training the young child, we should now be entering a golden age. The children so trained should now be flowering into free happy parenthood, founding united, creative, purposeful families. Maturity should have come to those trained in irresponsibility and given excuses for any character defects. They should be giving a fine burst of leadership to nations, with new and exciting purpose surging through politics, art and literature. The new insights should after a generation have given a new companionship and understanding between parents and children, youth and age. Our mental hospitals should be emptying; our suicide rates (one of the few quantitative tests) should be dropping year by year; aggression and violence should be more and more a thing of the past. Unity in the home and peace between nations should cover the earth. Is that what we see? If not, we must critically examine the philosophy which has shaped our contemporary scene.

Reluctant Reappraisement

For many working doctors this reappraisement was begun reluctantly. We did not want to surrender our 'Brave New World' and we did so unwillingly.

For some of us it was the results of analysis that raised our first doubts. Patients emerged self-centred, obsessed almost by the process they had gone through. Some told us that now they understood their internal conflicts and had accepted their reality; they had in some cases decided to live as sexual deviants or as men of lust, and having lost any deep sense of guilt, were now free. This did not seem like cure to us. An account published in the early thirties of a group of 'cured' patients who had committed suicide raised further doubts.

An additional factor in my own case was the reading of J. D. Unwin's *Sex and Culture*.[4] Unwin pointed out that according to Freud's theory of sublimation, there should be an inverse relation between sexual opportunity and the level of civilisation attained. In a monumental study of eighty primitive societies and six civilisations including our own he found that the stricter the sexual regulations, the higher the cultural level reached. 'Any society,' he said, 'is free to choose either to display great energy or to enjoy sexual freedom; the evidence is that it cannot do both for more than a generation.' (What price, then, our permissive society?) Aldous Huxley[2] says of Unwin's work, 'The evidence for these conclusions is so full that it is difficult to see how they can be rejected,' yet anthropologists have largely ignored them. What seemed to me very odd was that the psychologists also ignored them, and even seemed to regard sexual discipline as a dangerous practice, rather than as a means to intellectual and cultural achievement.

At this time the work of Ian Suttie[5] of the Tavistock Clinic brought a shaft of light. He showed how a man of such genius as Freud could be deceived on a matter so fundamental as the nature of love. Suttie's approach was objective. The facts, he believed, unlike material collected by analysis, could be seen and checked by several observers. He drew attention to the social aspects of love. He pointed out that even the child at the breast wants not only milk but unity with the mother. In that rapport lies security, born of affection and of response to it. From the earliest days, play, especially with the mother, but also with others in and around the family, develops security and the ability to receive and give love, and it is on this that maturity in great measure depends. Many of us would confirm that we too have seen and observed and experienced much of this. We are grateful to him for emphasising it.

Freud of course had never been 'in love', as he himself admits.[6] Is this why he is blind to the social and protective aspects of love and indeed to the whole non-sexual side? Eros he knew, Agape he never understood. May this also be the reason for his denigration of the mother's part in the family and of woman's in society?

As Suttie's work brought new illumination, Freud's continuing feud with Adler sowed further doubt. Could a really great scientist, a man whose field of study included man and his motives, be so vindictive and jealous? Could one who apparently understood so little of his own motives be so overwhelmingly right about those of others?

Glasser's Reality Therapy
We may find the clue in Ferenczi's well known statement:

'The physician's love heals the patient.' Recent work embodied in William Glasser's papers and his *Reality Therapy*[7] expand and amplify this. His conceptions are exciting and revolutionary. Consider this quotation: 'The therapist who accepts excuses, ignores reality, or allows the patient to blame his present unhappiness on a parent or on an emotional disturbance can usually make his patient feel good temporarily at the price of evading responsibility. He is only giving the patient 'psychiatric kicks' which are no different from the brief kicks he may have obtained from alcohol, pills or sympathetic friends before consulting the psychiatrist. When they fade, as they soon must, the patient, with good reason, becomes disillusioned with psychiatry.'

Where then does reality lie? Glasser maintains that a sense of worthwhileness is one major need and that this depends on standards of behaviour. The other major need is to love and accept love. Here he and Suttie closely agree.

Responsibility according to Glasser is 'the ability to fulfil our needs in a way that does not deprive others of the ability to fulfil theirs'. This involves right choice and right behaviour. When his patients blame circumstances or parents or childhood experiences, he says, 'All right, but in today's situation what are you going to do?' and again, 'Now you must by your right decision recover responsibility, break out of your self-centredness and step by step take on the world around.' Such ideas are very much in line with the experiences I have described earlier in this chapter, and indeed provide a rationale for them.

Glasser's results are encouraging and impressive. Taking patients already living in hospital for ten or fifteen years and condemned more or less for life, he has by graded responsibility week by week involved them more and more till they could emerge briefly on parole, then on probation and lastly return to society.

He stresses one important aspect. Patients, he says, always test the doctor's responsibility by asking for too much freedom too early. If he gives it, they say, 'He doesn't care. He doesn't love me.' If he refuses, they smile and say,

'You are right.' Does this restore some confidence to the parent in the home? Does it encourage him or her not to abdicate all authority and so forfeit their children's love? I think it does.

The great strength of this revolution of thought is that it can be immediately applied to the nation's life. It matches the basic beliefs of our religion. In an age of double talk and hypocrisy, this is important.

Honesty is central to reality therapy – total, absolute on the side of the therapist, and later accepted by the patient. But it is honesty with compassion. For this reason, Glasser takes Sir Thomas More in *A Man for All Seasons* as a true example of the therapeutic relationship. Henry VIII in the play wants Sir Thomas More to sanction and approve of his divorce. He wants this although he himself has power to sanction any divorce, even his own. When asked, 'Why?' he answers, 'Because you are honest'; because, in therapeutic terms, he wants to bolster up his sense of self-worth by the support of a man of undoubted integrity and honesty. Sir Thomas refuses. He cares enough for the King to risk all by his refusal to condone. Because they were personally deeply involved, the King now has to choose. He chooses irresponsibility and divorce, and turns against his Chancellor with deep bitterness and unjust criticism. Sir Thomas's execution follows. Fortunately, in hospital and usually in life, the therapist cannot be removed so easily.

Glasser, with many examples, traces how involvement, defined by him as care for some person or persons, begins cure. Deepening responsible behaviour follows, and gradually the patient's sense of self-worth increases and with it right behaviour. This is cure and leads to return to society and a full life. So successful has Glasser been that we must pay serious attention when he says, 'There is no such thing as mental disease. Only different ways of being irresponsible.'

Can we see in these conceptions something of value in the family, in the school and in the community? Can training and involvement begin early in life? It is popular to deny this. The idea is sedulously spread that a child of less than ten or twelve years cannot formulate moral judgements.

Few doctors will accept this and fewer parents. Indeed all who work with infants have learnt to sense in a baby's cry the difference between a genuine call for help and a selfish demand for attention. We also know that we can firmly yet lightheartedly show that we know the difference. At this age training in reality can begin.

Similarly, very early, a child can understand and accept an apology from a parent, with smiles succeeding tears, and guilt and restraint dispelled by an act of forgiveness. Very early, too, the child will test out each parent to try to make him or her behave irresponsibly. In this situation, Glasser states, 'The parents must understand that the child needs responsible parents and that taking the responsible course will never permanently alienate the child.' 'In essence,' he writes, 'we gain self respect through discipline and closeness to others through love.' These are statements many parents will welcome.

As in the home, so at school. If a child's ability to face life successfully depends on 'a series of personal involvements with responsible people', are not teachers among the most responsible he will meet, and do not doctors and nurses follow closely, with briefer but often crucial encounters? This attitude to education and training is optimistic, exciting and rewarding. As one who teaches each year 150 medical students and a goodly number of doctors, I see the same principles in action. Much of student activity today is a sophisticated testing of the authorities, tempting them to be irresponsible, and indeed the whole permissive cult is essentially the same thing. On the other hand, as responsibility is developed the mental climate in home, school and community begins to alter. A sense of self-worth grows and there is deepening and extending involvement in others.

If this is explored and applied, and if at the same time an answer is brought to fear, hate and greed, the age of cynicism in which we live may give place to a new age of participation, progress and fulfilment. Not only will family and national health improve with immense saving of time and money, but men and women will become truly free.

REFERENCES

(1) R. B. CATTELL: 'Scientific Analysis of Personality (Penguin, 1965), p. 17.

(2) ALDOUS HUXLEY: 'Ends and Means' (Chatto and Windus, 1937).

(3) ANNA FREUD: 'Normality and Pathology in Childhood' (Hogarth Press, 1966), pp. 5-8.

(4) J. D. UNWIN: 'Sex and Culture' (Oxford University Press, 1939). There is also a shorter book by Unwin, summarising his arguments, entitled 'Sexual Relations and Human Behaviour' (Williams and Norgate, 1933).

(5) IAN SUTTIE: 'Origin of Love and Hate' (Penguin, 1963).

(6) SIGMUND FREUD: 'Civilisation and its Discontents' (Hogarth Press, 1963,) p. 21.

(7) WILLIAM GLASSER: 'Reality Therapy' (Harper and Row, New York, 1965).

14

THE THEOLOGY OF SALVATION

The Rt. Rev. IAN THOMAS RAMSEY, D.D.,
Bishop of Durham

The Concept of Disclosure

Before discussing the theology of salvation as we find it in its classical expression in St Paul, I would like to say something in this introductory paragraph about a concept which is central to my exposition – the concept of self-discovery that I call elsewhere self-disclosure. I shall claim that the 'whole man' – this new 'creation' – is given in a self-discovery, or self-awareness, or self-disclosure, which occurs when subjectively I 'come to myself', when my public behaviour, or what is (or could be) known about me scientifically, takes on 'depth' or a 'new dimension'. But it is important from the outset to realise that self-disclosure occurs within a situation which comes alive objectively as well, where God discloses himself, a disclosure which for the Christian is of God's love in Christ. It has been said that the world's problems exist largely because of the nature and behaviour of the people that comprise it. What seems to me to be needed for genuine progress is the emergence of a 'new man', one who is being made 'whole' or is being 'healed' of his inadequacies by a response to God's love. History and scripture shows that such a man emerges in the first place through self-discovery. What a man can become is disclosed when he realises his own nature, catches a glimpse of this love and so is inspired and empowered to change.

To illustrate this concept of disclosure, let me begin with the story of David and Nathan and Nathan's use of the parable of the little ewe lamb. David, it will be remembered, had been moved by the beauty of his neighbour's wife

Bathsheba, and had arranged for her husband to be killed conveniently so that he could have her without embarrassing difficulties. Nathan tells the story of the little ewe lamb,* of the person who spared to take of his own flock when an unexpected guest arrived to dinner, but sent down the road and took the one ewe lamb of a poor family. David listens to the story; he pronounces judgment with force and emotion, and might have been said to be 'concerned' about the matter. But he had not 'come to himself', and only did so when the pattern of his own life 'clicked' with the parable which Nathan had told; when, as a result of a parable having the same form as, in other words being isomorphous with, the pattern of his own life, there was a self-disclosure and he knew that he was the man.

Another example may be taken from a more general context. We all know what happens when, after long deliberation, in a complicated situation, with many pros and cons, we suddenly 'see' our duty, and make what is the right moral decision, without fear or favour as it would be said. When such a duty or obligation is disclosed, when a man might remark with echoes of Luther, 'Here I stand and can no other,' then here we have a situation which is in principle all-inclusive in its character, where in principle everything else has been gathered in, and where the man, in making his decision, is confronted by, so to say, the whole universe. Here then is a cosmic disclosure which can be interpreted in terms of an encounter with God, and it is in such a discovery that a man comes to himself and knows his full subjectivity. Self-discovery, the emergence of that situation in which we aptly use first person assertions of affirmation and involvement, is no isolated, segregated occurrence. I come to myself as the world, as other people, come alive around me.

It may help to make the duty story clearer if I give one supplementary example of disclosures, with which indeed I might have introduced the discussion. Suppose we started to construct an unending series of regular polygons, so that their vertices were always equidistant from a certain fixed

* II Samuel 12, v. 1-7.

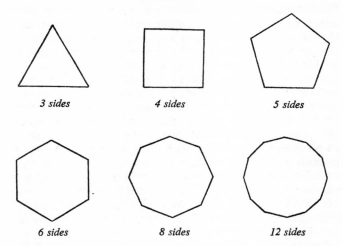

3 sides   4 sides   5 sides

6 sides   8 sides   12 sides

point. We would begin with a triangle, followed by a square, then by a pentagon, a hexagon, a heptagon, an octagon, a nonagon, a decagon and so on.

Suppose we repeated this process many times and then asked some observer at some particular stage what he saw. He might remark a polygon of (say) a thousand and four hundred and forty-four sides. In one sense he could be absolutely right. But we should know that the point of the game had not been taken. For we would hope that at some point or another around and by means of these regular polygons there might be disclosed something else, distinctively different from them all. We would hope for something we would call the disclosure of a circle. Sides, sides and more sides ... and at some point or another there might be disclosed a circle. So with the doctor, empirical events and more empirical events might, at some point or other, lead to a disclosure in which the doctor could come to himself and discern what was his particular duty on that particular occasion.

The Christian Concept of Salvation

Now let us turn to specifically Christian commitment, to

that 'coming to oneself' which is distinctly Christian. This arises as our appropriate response when a cosmic disclosure occurs, which in one way or another arises around the person of Jesus set in the pattern of his environment, his life and teaching, the crucifixion, Easter Day and so on. Christians in claiming Jesus as God and Man would further claim that in this particular cosmic disclosure there is only *one* individuation, that of God himself. The claim is that when the historical pattern, the 'Jesus of history', comes alive, the individuation like that of the universe, or that of an all-compelling duty, is the individuation of God. When in such a situation we come to ourselves, when in this situation a self-disclosure occurs and we 'come alive,' the phrase aptly used about us is that we have found 'eternal life in Christ Jesus our Lord'. This is not just healthy biological or psychological life nor is it just full economic, sociological or political life, though 'life eternal' is an existence which includes all such partial fulfilments. 'Life eternal' is not even 'dutiful life in response to some moral claim' though it includes this as well. It is even more than might be called 'immortality in God' for it is something that specifically involves Christ. It relates to a situation which is both subjectively and objectively distinctive, and which needs the distinctive phrase 'eternal life in Christ Jesus our Lord' as currency for it.

The Whole Man in St Paul's Writings

How far is this view of salvation with its stress on 'the whole person', foreign (say) to St Paul who, it might be said, seems to revel in a trichotomy – flesh (or body) mind and spirit – something even worse than Descartes with his dichotomy of mind and body.

Let us begin with reference to St Paul's discussion in Romans 8, and with his distinction there between 'flesh' and 'spirit', and similar themes in I and II Corinthians. Romans 8 might seem to the casual reader to suggest at least a dichotomy; in verse 4, he contrasts those who walk 'after the flesh', and those who 'walk after the spirit'. This contrast of verse 4 is emphasised even more strongly in verse 5. 'They that are after the flesh do mind (in other

170

words: seek, strive after, pursue) the things of the flesh, but they that are after the spirit, the things of the spirit.' Could there be, it might be asked, a plainer expression of a dichotomy between flesh and spirit, a parallel reminiscent of the dichotomy between body and mind?

But the contrast which St Paul is making is not one between mind and body, or between flesh and spirit thought of as dichotomous. The contrast is between on the one hand a person who makes his fleshly activities his dominant concern and pursuit, and on the other hand, a person who recognises that while he is fleshly he is also much more, and that he has an existence which while it certainly includes, also extends beyond his eating, drinking and reproductive functions. This wider existence in which a man is fulfilled, in which he finds his 'wholeness' or 'salvation' is an existence which is revealed, which he finds in a self-disclosure, when he knows God and God's power and love in Jesus Christ. One man seeks and strives after eating, drinking and a colourful and satisfying social existence; he has a mind and a concern for nothing else and his end, his final goal is, consistently enough, death. 'The mind of the flesh is death' (Romans 8, v. 6). Another man may seek and strive after eating, drinking and a colourful and vigorous social life, but does not set these as his goal. He eats, drinks and reproduces, he is ill and of course he dies like the rest, but the very frailty, the very transitoriness and the very imperfections which belong to all these 'fleshly' activities, become occasions for discovering and making plain the fuller life of the spirit. His dominant loyalty to God's love in Christ constantly transforms his eating, drinking, reproducing, being ill and even dying. The one may be a whole man, but his integration comes from a purpose which is entirely earthly-centred. The other is a whole man with an integration which comes from a purpose which arises in a situation of a transcendent kind, transcendent, that is, in not being restricted to the spatio-temporal elements of which scientific discourse speaks.

If it is complained that this is an excessive interpretation to put on a few verses from Romans 8, let us look at the same theme as it arises in another epistle, I Corinthians.

Here the contrast is not between those who 'walk after the flesh' and those who 'walk after the spirit'; now it is between the 'natural' man and the 'spiritual' man. The natural man (I Corinthians 2, v. 14), we shall not be surprised to hear, is the man 'who receiveth not the things of the spirit of God'. Such things are 'foolishness unto him', they are fatuous, vacuous, empty, because he is concerned with only what can be seen, heard, touched, tasted and smelt. But the spiritual man, we are told, 'examineth all things'. He takes everything into consideration, he has a wider assessment, and the implication is that he recognises the 'deep things of God'. The same distinction lies behind St Paul's treatment of the resurrection in chapter 15 of the same epistle. Man begins as the first Adam and the word 'Adam' is closely related to the Hebrew word for earth. Man begins as these and those molecules, with a natural personality and a natural life. The Christian gospel is not a message of denial, it is rather a message of transformation which tells of how this 'natural' personality can become 'spiritual', so that Adam is given a new life. 'If any man is in Christ, he is a new creature' (II Corinthians 5, v. 17, c.p. Galatians 6, v. 15), there is a new creation, a second Adam, a new fulfilment of personality. This is the Christian person 'made whole'.

We may remark how very easily St Paul's thinking develops out of his Jewish background. Semitic influences were already there, and the Old Testament always viewed man as a whole, man as a unity. In Genesis 2, v. 7, which was expressly in St Paul's mind in I Corinthians 15, we read, 'The Lord God formed man of the dust of the ground, and breathed into his nostrils the breath of life, and man became a living soul', and the Hebrew word there is 'Nepesh', a breathing, living thing, a person or a self, something which we can translate at will, 'soul', 'spirit', 'mind', 'person' – Hebrew has no significant distinction. All that mattered was that the breathing through this unitary organism should be God's breathing, that the breath, the 'ruach', should be the spirit of God. Here was the first creation, the natural man, and when God acted in Christ there was, so to say, a second in-breathing. Whereas the first gave a man human life, his natural personality, the second gave him eternal life, his Christian status. The first gave man the status of a creature, the second redeemed him. But the important point is that both concerned his whole personality; both concerned him as a unity. The first in-breathing made man, as a creature, distinctive, superior to the animals for example; he was made in the image of God. Then came what is called 'The Fall'. The second in-breathing made him a new creature, a creature for a second time; the likeness, the image was restored. This may be a picturesque, quasi-historical account of the nature of man; but for our present purpose the important point is that from first to last man is conceived as a unity.

We may well admit that St Paul did sometimes speak of man as though he were a dichotomy or a trichotomy, body and spirit, or mind and spirit, or flesh and spirit, or body, mind and spirit. I am quite clear further, that Paul's phrases could mislead, and have misled for instance such a one as Apollinarius who misunderstood a verse at the end of the first letter to the Thessalonians where Paul speaks of preserving 'Spirit and soul and body ... entire' (I Thess. 5, v. 23). But Apollinarius was a heretic and should be a warning and not an example to follow. St Paul never wrote, let us remember, as an analytic philosopher. He had, for better or worse (we might well think for better) no cut and dried metaphysics. What he used were concepts which, while they could be misunderstood if they brought with them too much of a metaphysical background, were only being used by him as vehicles for expressing a doctrine of salvation which unquestionably concerned the whole man. When St Paul was concerned to express fully, and in its most general form, the Christian doctrine of man he uses, as we have seen, language which is independent of any trichotomous or dichotomous expressions. There is on the one hand the natural man, human personality with all its functions, living in the maximum independence of and in due course, not surprisingly, in enmity to God. With that 'natural' man St Paul contrasts the 'spiritual' man whose total personality is 'in Christ' and who, being open to the influence of God in Christ, is a new creation. To St Paul then, he who is in Christ, he who is redeemed and sanctified, is a new creature who has found life and peace. He it is in totality who is spiritual, and 'spiritual' in that sense means that his whole personality is influenced and transformed by the love of God in Christ, which then characterises all his relationships and not least those of the flesh. Whatever this man does, whether he eats, drinks, or reproduces, he does all to the glory of God. He is a whole man indeed.

We need not deny that many of his successors fathered on Paul a flesh/spirit dualism which, further, would regard the flesh as essentially wicked and the spirit alone as good. But we must remember that such exaggerations characterise not orthodoxy but heresy, not reliable thinking, but mistaken thinking – heresies known to text books as gnosticism, manicheism, montanism, docetism and the rest, heresies which in one way or another, give an admittedly incomplete account of the redemption which is in Christ.

Implications for Science and Medicine

Before coming to my concluding section, there is another point I might usefully make. Contemporary theology, as much as contemporary philosophy and medicine, works in terms of the concept of the whole personality rather than with (say) mind and body thought of as a dichotomy. But for the Christian, the 'whole man', the new creation, is a person who has 'come to himself' by responding to the saving word and work of Christ; and this newness of life will be spelt out, but never exhaustively given, in biological and other strands throughout the whole of a man's life. Here is a self-disclosure which cannot be adequately treated in scientific discourse without denying the very subjectivity, the very first person ('subject') discourse which all scientific discourse about 'objects' presupposes.

My broad conclusion then is this. We come to ourselves as 'whole persons' when we realise our full personalities in times of self-discovery, and to evoke such self-disclosure must be the aim of all scientific and medical skills and knowledge used in a humane context. What contemporary discoveries in science show, whether in neuro-surgery, cybernetics, biochemistry, or elsewhere, is that the situations in which this subjectivity is realised are rapidly becoming vastly different from any we have known before. But disclosures of subjectivity will still be logically possible, and they will always be morally significant. Scientific 'explanations' of the self or human behaviour will never exclude other 'explanations' in a different logical key. People will only be 'cured' if they are enabled to 'come to themselves', in disclosure situations, Christian or other. At this point, however, I seem to be forced to a conclusion which I realise is medically often unpopular. If religious language and ministrations work at the disclosure level, then we cannot deny *some* kind of link between this language and these ministrations on the one hand, and biochemistry, psychiatry and so on, on the other. I do *not* say that conclusions about a man's health or his biochemistry or his psychological health will ever be *deduced* from theological assertions. But we must not conclude from this that theological assertions and religious ministrations are then empirically irrelevant. All that follows is that they will follow no stereotyped, easily predictable pattern. But empirical correlates we must believe that they do have.

Self-examination and Self-denial

Having reached that unpopular conclusion on the medical side, let me make one which may be equally unpopular on the theological side. What I have called self-discovery and 'self-knowledge' must be severely distinguished from the 'self-examination' of a traditional kind, though in fairness we must recognise that at best such self-examination was meant to reveal God as a preliminary to a disclosure of ourselves.

The same point might be made about self-denial. Self-denial is never to be commended by the Christian, or anyone else, for its own sake. To deny the self *in vacuo* is as much mistaken as to assert it in an isolated selfishness. It is of course a very different matter to lose a life 'for my sake and the Gospel's.' For this is to find a life, a fulfilment, by responding to that disclosure of God's love around Christ which is the Gospel. What we undoubtedly need in our own time are first, disciplines and procedures, whether in theology or medicine, which lead reliably to self-discovery, disclosure of the fulfilling, all-embracing, transforming kind which I have been at pains to elucidate, and then, secondly, conceptual schemes, whether in medicine or theology, adequate and appropriate to talk of what happens.

The Social Dimension

I realise that in this paper so far I have not done anything like justice to the social dimension of salvation. So let me conclude by remedying somewhat this inadequacy.

Just as the self revealed in the subjectivity of a disclosure situation, is more than the aggregate of all the aspects of all the different scientific strands that are relevant to it, so in a parallel way those who practise these different disciplines in order that the patient may 'come alive', may be brought to self disclosure, healing and salvation – these people will discover their fellowship together in a true community as and when their different disciplines combine creatively in that disclosure situation or 'rebirth' which embraces doctor as well as patient. The patient 'comes alive', rediscovers 'himself' as the 'whole man', the man who is 'healed' and 'saved', in a context which is then both secular and Christian, and this context is one where those who minister the different healing techniques may themselves, like the patient, come alive. In their case this will then be to form a true healing community.

In other words, if the whole man, the man who is saved and healed, has found his wholeness, salvation, healing in a disclosure, we have a situation in which a social dimension will have been given at the same time to medicine itself, for around and integrating medical practice will have been disclosed true fellowship, characterising a community. So the therapeutic, healing community is the correlate of the whole person, as the Church is the correlate of the redeemed Christian. A specifically Christian hospital does its work in relation to the 'saving work of

Christ, disclosure-given'. But because this is a revelation, given in this way, it is difficult to speak of such a hospital except in elusive and allusive phrases like 'atmosphere'. There can be no question of 'imposing' a Christian vision, compelling Christian healing, any more than we can compel someone to see a joke. All we can do is to set the Christian gospel before people, and proclaim the saving work of Christ, so that those whom we serve will respond spontaneously to find healing and salvation, and a newness of life that finds progressive fulfilment; a new creation, 'eternal life in Christ Jesus our Lord'.

This paper is essentially a modified version of part of a paper already published in a symposium entitled *The Whole Man* and is reproduced by permission of the editor, Dr. J. McGilvray.

Conclusion

15

CURING A SICK SOCIETY

GARTH LEAN, M.A.

*Garth Lean is the author of "John Wesley, Anglican",
and of "Brave Men Choose", short biographies of men
who have applied Christianity in British politics in
the last two centuries. With Sir Arnold Lunn, he has
also written two best-selling books of religious controversy,* The New Morality *and* The Cult of Softness.
*This chapter touches on ideas developed more fully
by him in their third book,* Christian Counter-Attack.

Each in his own way, the distinguished contributors to this
book have pursued the themes of health, of character and
morals, and of the nature of society. And in the writing the
three themes have merged into one.

Society impinges on the individual at so many points that
individual health can no longer be guaranteed in an unhealthy society. Contrariwise, as Alice would say, only
healthy individuals – people healthy in body, mind and
spirit – can make a really healthy society. So whether we are
considering with Dr McKay how to stop the destruction of
our environment or noting with Dr Metcalfe Brown that
many of the regress points in national health go back to
places where individual men fail in wisdom or self-discipline, we are led back to the importance of individual character. 'Most of us enjoy good physical health', writes Dr
Brown, 'but what of spiritual health? "We have left undone those things which we ought to have done. And we
have done those things which we ought not to have done.

178

And there is no health in us." If this is true, the remedy for the nation is in the hands of the nation.'

The Search for a New Type of Man

In fact, the curing of a sick society – and many will agree with Dr Keele that ours is 'very sick' – depends on making bad people good and good people better on a massive scale. Here our contributors are on common ground with those who think our Western society sickest – with the various revolutionaries who think it so sick, indeed, that it must be destroyed and rebuilt from the bottom up. For all real revolutionaries look for salvation to the production of a new and better kind of human being – and the revolutionaries of today are no exception. This is as true of the new style revolutionaries of Student Power and Black Power as it is of the old-style Communists of Russia.

Lenin thought that the new conditions under Communism would produce a new human being who would naturally work for the community rather than for himself. But fifty years have passed since the Russian revolution and the new man seems as far away in the future as ever. A founder of the Norwegian Communist Party, Hans Bjerkholt, once told me that the question of this new type of man was the 'unfinished business' at every Moscow conference he attended – unfinished because it remained a theory which never became a fact. In his brilliant novel, *Cancer Ward*[1] – a book which will particularly interest doctors – Alexander Solzhenitsyn makes the old Bolshevik, Shulubin, say: 'We thought it was enough to change the mode of production and immediately people would change as well. But did they change? The hell they did! They didn't change a bit.'

The apostles of student power, who look to China and Cuba rather than to Russia, also seek a new type of man. Neal Ascherson summarised their aims and aspirations perceptively in *The Observer* shortly after the Paris days of May 1968. After discussing the influence of Professor Marcuse and Che Guevara, of Chairman Mao and psychologist Wilhelm Reich, he continued:

The professor and the guerrilla, the chairman and the

psychologist, are illustrations to a revolutionary text which – allowing for different traditions – reads much the same wherever the young go on the street. Parliaments are moribund; liberalism is a dangerous sham concealing the most efficient repression ever known. Moscow and Washington are power bureaucracies, brainwashing their masses by a manipulated Press into believing they are content. Society should be run by spontaneous workers' councils, by continuous democracy. Capitalism leads these days towards a sort of technocratic Fascism (and French and German students believe that Mr Wilson demonstrates this): it must go. Then a new human being will arise: unexploited, creative in the leisure granted by automation, spontaneous, uninhibited, social. And, if the truth be told, it is this New Adam who is the only hero the students really worship.[2]

Alas, neither the New Adam, nor the new society springs so automatically from the destruction of an old order. If a new and better type of man had in fact already been produced, one could hope that a new and better society might follow. But the student activists have not yet convinced even their own generation that they have developed the character necessary to underwrite a beneficial revolution. A party of young Czechs who visited the student leader Rudi Dutschke in Berlin in the spring of 1967 reported back: 'There was no contact. People like Dutschke think they are talking about revolutionary democracy. If they had their way it would lead to Stalinism again.'[3]

Similarly, Franz Fanon, the black psychiatrist from Martinique, whose book *The Wretched of the Earth*[4] is said to be the bible of the Black Power movement, cried: 'For Europe, for ourselves and for humanity, comrades, we must turn a new leaf, we must work out new concepts, and try and set afoot a new man.' 'These are brave and challenging words', commented Dr Martin Luther King. 'But the problem is that Fanon and those who quote his words are seeking to "work out new concepts" and "set afoot a new man" with a willingness to imitate old concepts of violence. Is not there a basic contradiction here?

Violence has been the inseparable twin of materialism, the hallmark of its grandeur and misery. This is the one thing about modern civilization that I do not care to imitate.'[5]

Solzhenitsyn's Shulubin says much the same, 'You can't have a socialism that's always banging on about hatred,' he tells his fellow patient in the cancer ward. 'After a man burns with hatred, year in, year out, he can't simply announce one fine day, 'That's enough. As from today I'm finished with hatred, from now on I'm only going to love." No, if he's used to hating he'll go on hating. He'll find someone closer to him whom to hate.'

Christian Revolution

Is there a way of improving man which is more successful than the way of hatred? Many of the contributors in this book suggest that this is best achieved through religion – and imply that it is vitally necessary if men or society are to be healed. Dr Lambourne, for example, reminds us that the pre-war tendency to trust to technology and the welfare state at the expense of 'voluntary caring' has now been reversed and concludes by emphasising the unique part which dedicated Christian individuals and groups can play. The Bishop of Durham sees the heart of the matter in 'a new creation' where the individual 'responds spontaneously to find the healing and salvation and newness of life which finds progressive fulfilment'. The Archbishop of Canterbury put it more directly in an address to students at the London School of Economics. 'Christianity,' he said, 'is the most revolutionary creed in the world because it seeks a revolution in man himself.'[6]

The distinctive fact about Christianity is that it not only seeks such a revolution, but achieves it. Wherever Christianity is lived out without compromise or hold-back, lives change. The lives of the saints are not the only evidence of this. Wesley's work, according to the historian, J. H. Overton, 'made the selfish man self-denying, the discontented happy, the worldling spiritually-minded, the drunkard sober, the sensual chaste, the liar truthful, the thief honest, the proud humble, the godless godly, the thriftless thrifty'.[7]

And these new men did much to cure a sick society. Most historians agree that it was the change in thousands of ordinary British people which made possible the great social reforms of the nineteenth century – the abolition of the slave trade and slavery, the reform of the prisons and factories, the start of general education and the fact that the British Labour movement developed with a mainly Christian, rather than a Marxist philosophy. Such people were the foot-soldiers of reform, but the leaders, too – William Wilberforce, Lord Shaftesbury and Keir Hardie to name only three – underwent the same transforming experience.

When Wilberforce, who was Pitt's best friend and might have been his successor, began his Parliamentary career, his 'own distinction' was, in his own words, his 'darling object'. After his change he wrote in his journal 'God Almighty has set before me two great objects, the suppression of the slave trade and the reformation of manners.'[8] It can truly be said that he did much to cure a sick society, for before his death both of these objects had, in large measure, been achieved. Without the deep changes in his own life, he would have been powerless to give such leadership. John Morley, in his life of Edmund Burke, wrote that Burke thought of taking up the fight for the abolition of the slave trade, but judged it beyond his scope. 'He was quite right,' commented Morley, 'in refusing to hope from any political action what could only be effected after moral preparation of the bulk of the nation – and direct apostleship was not his function.'.[9] Wilberforce, following his conversion, was better equipped – and the tens of thousands who had found a faith through the Evangelical Revival were there to play their part. Politics is said to be 'the art of the possible', but these men made possible in their day what had been impossible a few years before. This is the statesmanship of Christianity in every age.

Fresh Hope for the World

Can an individual change still bring healing to society in this complicated, technological age? Mr Alan Thornhill, in his contribution to this book, describes how the change in a dockers' leader brought healing to the dock industry of his city. If further evidence is needed, one has only to turn to a book like Gabriel Marcel's *Un Changement d'Espérance à la Rencontre du Réarmement Moral*, published in this country by Longmans, Green under the title *Fresh Hope for the World.* M. Marcel who is one of France's most distinguished philosophers and playwrights, there sets out sixteen examples out of 'a hundred known to him'. They include the French Socialist leader who was freed from her hatred of the Germans and then played a significant part in bringing about the reconciliation of France and Germany during the fifties, the textile employer and the national trades union secretary whose transformed attitudes led to the French textile agreement which M. Pinay hailed as the model for all France, the Brazilian dockers who abandoned gang warfare and introduced the first democratic union to the docks of Rio de Janeiro, and a dozen others. In answer to the objection that individual changes are too simple a method in our complicated modern society, M. Marcel writes:

To my mind simplicity is a positive quality – the value of which goes almost entirely unrecognised in a world like ours that is on the verge of losing itself in its own complexity. One ought, really, to think out carefully which are the spheres where complexity is inevitable and the price of any real progress – and where it is literally disastrous and could even be said to checkmate itself. Whereever technique is supreme – and I am thinking especially of the technique needed to help forward man's operations on nature – it is hard to see how one can avoid complexity; indeed complexity seems to be the only way to achieve the ever greater precision that is necessary. This complexity applies both to the calculations and to the instruments that are made possible and efficient by these calculations. But the extraordinary thing, which very few people realise, is that the moment you enter the realm of the *human* everything becomes different. ... The moment you say this ... you cease to think of a man as a machine. You will realize the importance of this if you recall that for my friends the fundamental experience is one of change, not just a subjective change, but a radical change of the personality.[10]

Medical men have an unique opportunity to initiate such 'radical changes of personality' in this age, for they have largely taken the place, formerly held by the parson or even the parent, of being the recipient of difficult confidences. No more than any other Christians can they impose their vision on those who come to them, but many may – as the Bishop of Durham writes – 'spontaneously' respond to their faith, provided it is real. For faith, like influenza, is infectious. And doctors, as I have found to my own profit, can pass on a more fundamental cure than aspirin or penicillin, a cure which can reach out through individuals to a larger world.

REFERENCES

(1) ALEXANDER SOLZHENITSYN: 'Cancer Ward' (Bodley Head, Part I 1968, Part II 1969).

(2) *The Observer*, 2 June 1968.

(3) *The Weekend Telegraph*, 6 December, 1968.

(4) FRANZ FANON: 'The Wretched of the Earth' (Penguin, 1967).

(5) MARTIN LUTHER KING: 'Chaos and Community' (Hodder and Stoughton, 1968), pp. 65-6.

(6) *The Times*, 21 November, 1968.

(7) J. H. OVERTON: 'The Evangelical Revival in the Eighteenth Century' (Longmans, 1886), p. 131.

(8) GARTH LEAN: 'Brave Men Choose' (Blandford, 1961), pp. 7-8.

(9) JOHN MORLEY: 'Edmund Burke: a Historical Study' (Macmillan, 1867).

(10) GABRIEL MARCEL: 'Fresh Hope for the World' (Longmans, 1960), pp. 4-5.